OneBody
Massage

Dedicated to the ones we hold dear to our hearts.

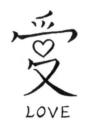

LOVE

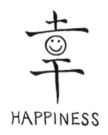

HAPPINESS

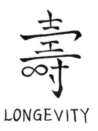

LONGEVITY

CONTENTS

WARNING!

We chose to use all capital letters to get your attention and let you know we are serious about insisting that you check in with your doctor before practicing any massage techniques described in this book. So please, for Pete's sake (my editor Pete Danko), ask your doctor if it is safe for you to give and receive massage. And keep in mind the importance of always checking often with the receiver of massage to make sure the level of pressure you are applying is appropriate. When in doubt, do not attempt a given technique.

ONE • ELEMENTS

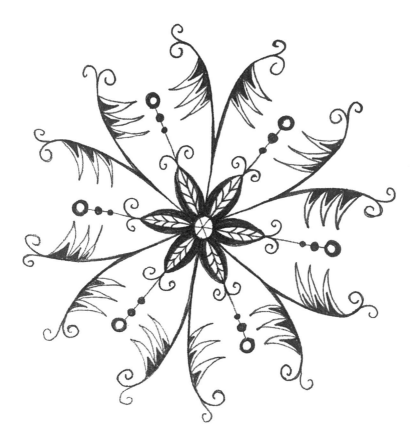

1

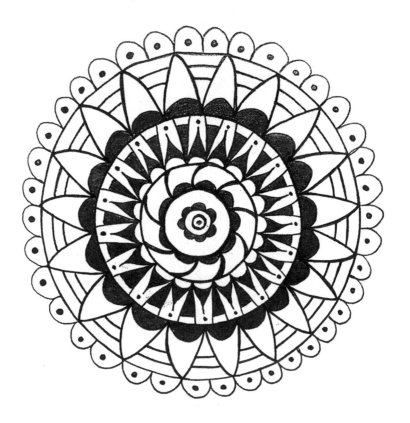

'If you are irritated by every rub, how
will your mirror be polished?'
~ Rumi~

The thing about working as a Web and graphic designer is that you sit on your ass a lot. I mean a lot. Staring countless hours into the monitor and fixing images to perfection pixel by pixel is not for the faint of heart. Sore eyes, neck and, shoulder, and back tension are the norm. Or so it seems. I know I didn't know what I was eating half of the time during my working lunches; once, I even found tiny green critters in my Caesar salad after I had already finished half of it! OK, so that was me back in the year 2000 working long hours under extremely tight deadlines. I ignored my discomfort because I believed it came with the job. No one else was complaining. So I buried my nose in my work, believing that the deadlines and stress were good because

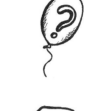
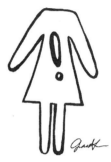

they made me more productive. Thanks to my strict Taiwanese Catholic upbringing, my mind was completely separated from my feelings and my body.

One day for a special event the company brought in a massage therapist to give each of us a twenty-minute chair massage. I was elated to have someone take care of my body. I shook the therapist Mike's hand and hopped on this odd-looking "chair." It was like riding a soft, padded horse with a face cradle. Within a minute I was out. I might not have snored, but I definitely drooled. At some point, Mike asked if I liked how much massage

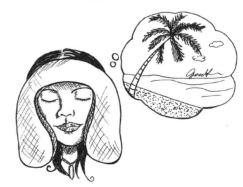

4

pressure he was using on me. I nodded and mumbled. I was in heaven. My body and mind both took a trip to La-La Land until a quiet voice called me back to reality.

"It feels like your neck tension travels all the way down to your upper back. And your forearms could use more stretching," Mike said.

I couldn't believe it. A complete stranger knew more about my body than I did! Something had to change – and I knew it. Somewhere in my subconscious mind I had been busy planning how, where and what I was going to do to get my foot into the realm of the healing arts. I was cautious. I did not dive headlong into the massage world by changing my lifestyle right away. I still went out and partied, returning home half-conscious to watch *The Simpsons* and eat Honey Flakes at two in the morning. Sometimes for kicks my husband, Ryan, and his cousin Brandon and I would make coffee shakes, French toast and bacon instead of Honey Flakes. We called it "Heart Attack on a Little Plate." Clotted arteries and high blood pressure didn't seem like a threat to us. It was cool to be defiant, to swear, to not care for our bodies as long as we could have "intellectual" conversations. Our cool act had many side effects, such as Brandon's morning headaches, Ryan's upset stomachs and my irritable temper. To mask our physical and emotional discomfort we would party even harder.

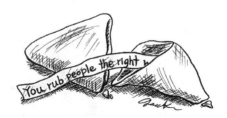

Remember my subconscious mind? She was secretly infiltrating my lifestyle by putting inspirational people in front of my face. One night, Ryan and I went out for Chinese food and the message in my fortune cookie read, "You rub people the right way." I guess if I were a character in a movie that would be considered foreshadowing. I went on to meet Jenny Shults, who was a chiropractor and homeopath. Her calming energy and knowledge of the body intrigued me. She used applied kinesiology and muscle testing to check which part of my body needed help. She asked me to stand up, raise my left arm and resist her pressure of pushing my arm down. It was easy. But when she asked me to turn my head to the right, my arm was quickly pushed down.

"What happened?" I asked her with astonishment. "How come my arm suddenly went weak?"

She said the brain is like the motherboard, sending out electrical signals to the body, but sometimes due to diet, posture or emotional imbalance the signals get confused. She checked the alignment of my neck and upper back. They were both out. As I was lying on the adjustment table facing up, the skylight created a halo effect over her long, flowing brown hair and I thought, "Wow, I want to be a modern witch like her." After she adjusted me she gave me some homeopathic remedies to help with my stress. What a nice witch!

She explained to me the concept of holistic health care, "holistic" meaning seeing a person on all levels: mental, emotional, physical and spiritual. All as one and one as all. When one element is out of balance the rest will be. So treating a person's physical discomfort, his obvious symptom like, say, neck pain, can offer some relief but may not heal him completely. The neck pain may in fact be connected to an emotional cause – a traumatic childhood experience, perhaps, like an angry father grabbing his neck when he did not perform well academically. Now, as an adult, threats of inadequacy could trigger the neck pain. In theory, healing him from the inside out and outside in will help him to identify the emotional trigger, to learn ways to recognize it and use easy, accessible techniques like breathing or meditation to control his feelings in a positive way. Other changes might include consuming food consciously, exercising regularly to help support and strengthen the neck muscles to increase flexibility, or applying massage and chiropractic therapy when needed. Ultimately, holistic healing enables people to be in charge of their own health. It helps them understand ways to listen to their bodies. The body speaks. If we quiet our mind, we can hear its wisdom.

A couple of months later I went on a business trip with Ryan to Venice Beach. While he worked I sat under a palm tree, sipping a glass of lemonade, scribbling away on a sketch pad, watching a shop owner make a deal with a tourist on a tie-dye Doors T-shirt. A strange man with two little white dogs approached me. The man asked if I could watch his dogs while he went to get them some water. "Sure, why not. I am on vacation." I gladly accepted the responsibility of watching two cuties. When the strange man returned with water he introduced himself and proceeded to share his story. Larry was his name. He was in his late fifties and worked as a clairvoyant energy healer. "A little strange," I thought to myself. Larry began to have visions when he was seven, seeing or sensing things that were not there, feeling what was about to happen. He lived with his single mother, who asked him to keep his "gift" a secret. He honored her request and went on living like a normal person until he had a midlife crisis, at which point he decided he was old enough to know what was best for himself. So he embraced his ability to sense and work with people's energy to help them heal. He told me his story, and then offered to check my energy balance for me.

"The strange man is offering to do energy work on me," I thought. "Should I let him?"

I looked around – people were biking and walking nearby. I figured I was safe. If anything got weird I could always yell out, "Fire!" Plus, I was on vacation, – there was nowhere I needed to be and nothing needed to be done.

"OK, sounds good," I told him.

Larry asked me to sit comfortably and look out to the ocean. First he did some massage to loosen up my shoulders, focusing on specific shoulder joints with a combination of rubbing, pulling and rotating. Then he reminded me to breathe. I took some deep breaths and felt a little bit more comfortable, like I was sitting more relaxed and taller at the same time. I felt this heat coming out of his hands on my lower back without him actually touching my back. It was soothing. He asked if I had ever injured my lower back. I told him when I was five I pretended to be Superman, red cape and all, and riding my tricycle as fast as I could, I took off from the top of the staircase. The next thing I knew I was crying for Mommy. Since then I've always had issues with my lower back and my right shoulder. Larry was concentrating on "moving blocked energy," as he called it, from my lower back. I felt the heat flowing from my lower back to the middle of my back and slowly spreading out to my shoulders and cooling off. It was a sense of relief, like finally letting go of a burden I had been carrying for a long, long while. I sighed and felt like crying. It was so good to be free of my emotional baggage. That was the first time I experienced how emotion is intertwined with the physical body. All thanks to Larry, a complete stranger who wanted nothing from me but half an hour of my time to heal me. Thank you, Larry, wherever you are.

My unexpected encounters with Jenny and Larry fueled my desire to learn more about the healing arts. The first massage class I took was shiatsu at Body Therapy Center in Palo Alto in 2003. Rachel Johnson, a calm English lady with short curly hair, knelt in front of the classroom and invited the whole class to sit on the floor.

"Be a free and relaxed wanderer," she told us. (This is the translation of a herbal remedy for the liver, "Hsaio Yao Wan.")

We started with breathing and stretching exercises, and discussed the theory of Eastern energetic body flow. The class was in the evening and was a great way to unwind after working all day. The best thing about massage class is that all of the students get to practice on each other. I was hooked. I wanted to learn more ways to work with the body.

In acupressure class, a more complex Chinese body system was introduced. The twelve meridians, energy pathways made with as many as two thousand acupuncture points, correlate to the five elements: wood, earth, water, metal, fire. Each element governs different emotions, seasons, senses, foods, colors, sounds and organs. Janet Oliver would explain the relationships between the elements – they were as confusing as trying to understand a foreign soap opera!

We also learned to listen to the wrist pulse, and study the tongue and the skin to determine which meridian might be out of balance. For example, the stomach and spleen correspond to the earth element, their color is yellow, the voice has a singing quality, their season is late summer, their emotion is

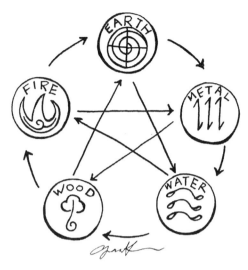

empathy, they govern the intellect and their sound association is "whooo." The earth element controls the water element and is controlled by the wood element. She mentioned that in ancient China, a physician only got paid when his patients were healthy. What a new way to think of health care!

Carol Fitzgerald, a relaxation massage teacher, liked to recite poetry at the beginning of each class. I can still hear her rhythmic voice – coupled with the silver bangles on her wrist – reciting Plato, "Be kind, for everyone you meet is fighting a hard

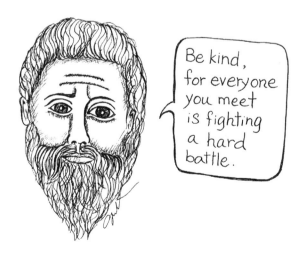

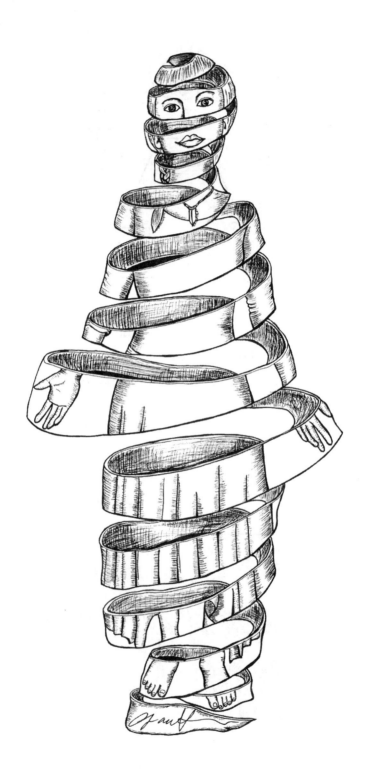

battle." We all have the capacity to practice compassion when we are reminded just how similar we all are. I was fortunate to take Upledger's SomatoEmotional Release class with Tim Hutton. He demonstrated the massage protocol technique and ways to dialogue with the body to help unwind both the somatic and emotional aspects. During the workshop, I could see receivers' bodies moving at different paces and in different directions. Some were quiet while others were crying or yelling. Tim also encouraged the class to trust our intuition. By listening with our hands and eyes in a massage session, we can tune in to the micro movements of the person we are touching, both physically

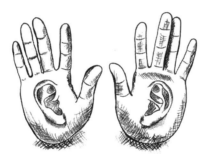

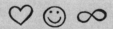

Trick of the Trade

**How to Switch to the Right Mind
for Giving a Massage**

We are complicated creatures by design, with many layers of emotion. Often we are not consciously aware of "ourselves," therefore it is not surprising we get distracted easily. To be the giver of massage, we practice compassion by clearing our thoughts and worries and setting a positive affirmation for the session without attachment to a particular outcome. Affirmation directs our intention toward positive change. I find that a simple mantra such as "May love and light shine through me, may love and light shine through you," works well to shift my mind to the right place. I focus on my breath whenever my mind starts to wonder, and the breath helps to pull me back into the center, into the present moment. Detachment from the outcome takes away my personal fixed view on how things should be, how my partner should feel, and provides a neutral ground for my partner's own healing expression.

and energetically. Instead of following specific massage steps we create a space for exploration and connection. He reminded us that a therapist should be nonjudgmental, ego-subordinated and unconditionally present. Not an easy task. I am still constantly reminding myself to be present, to follow my client's lead, and not to be attached to the outcome of the session.

Rachel and I met again nine years later in a Thai massage workshop. She began and ended every day with this simple prayer: "Be well, be safe, and be peaceful." (This is from the Buddhist principle of Metta Loving-Kindness, said as an affirmation about oneself, "May I be well, may I be safe, may I be peaceful, may I be happy," and then extended farther and farther out in any way you like from what is close and known, to what is remote.)

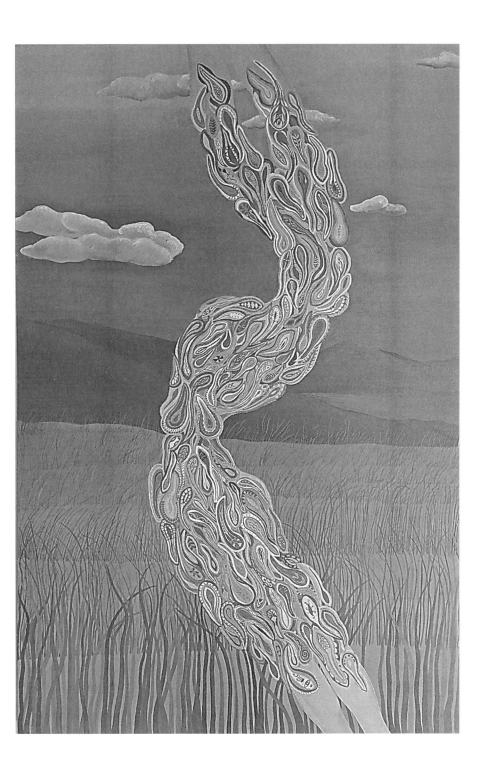

I have adopted her prayer into my own practice. The fortune cookie was right about my journey to happiness. I have met so many incredible teachers in the last decade of practicing massage, and some of the greatest teachers were my clients. Each client is unique, and the same client is different each time. Each massage practice deepens my appreciation of the human body which strives for function and equilibrium in a frequently imbalanced system. We find ways to move our body while compensating for injury, scar tissue or emotional blockage, all without knowing it. That realization amazes me. And it makes me humble. Every massage session is an opportunity to be in a calm, peaceful, suspended space where one is enveloped between heaven and earth, connecting with another. It's beautiful.

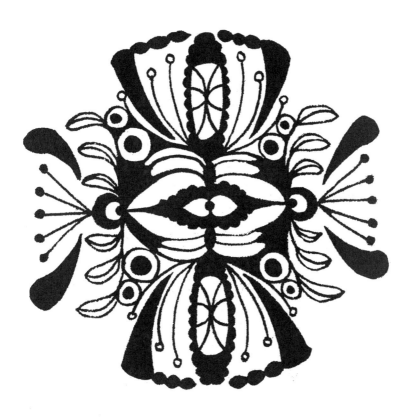

2

How are you feeling in your body today?

When a client walks into the massage room at Google to see me, I always begin with a question: "How are you feeling in your body today?" You would be amazed how often the answers start with, "I think." But my question is about *feeling*. People can't help themselves. In a fast-paced problem-solving Silicon Valley work environment like Google, people tend to think more than feel. My challenge as a massage therapist is to help my clients focus on what's going on in their body. I see people raising their shoulders to their ears, overextending their neck, shoulders rolled in towards their chest, typing with overextended wrists, sitting on their lower back, standing with their knees locked, breathing only with their upper chest. Maybe you think better while in an odd body position, but over time, the wear and tear on the muscles and joints starts to show. And the scary part is, even when you don't intend to sit or stand in an odd position the body often has a "mind" of its own. The body goes into that position by default.

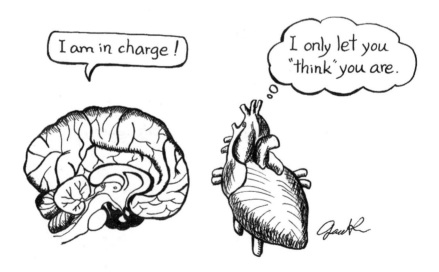

Neck, shoulder, back, wrist and forearm tension is so rampant in the workplace that at Google, an innovative company, besides offering massage, we have a team of chiropractors, physical therapists, personal trainers, ergonomic specialists and doctors to help Googlers with their wellness. For the rest of the world we have ourselves, friends and loved ones to keep us in line. As I am saying this to you, I am noticing I am wearing my left shoulder like an earring, pressed up to the side of my face, due to my habit of carrying my three-year-old in that arm. My jaw is clenched, which also causes my temporal lobes to tighten up. I am also putting a lot of tension between my eyebrows – *hmmm* – creating unnecessary wrinkles. So I remember my tai chi teacher Steven Cardoza's instruction on aligning my shoulders with my hips, resting the tip of my tongue on the roof of my mouth, imagining there is a string on top of my head that is pulling me toward the sky, and relaxing my forehead. Ah, those simple adjustments help me feel more comfortable in my own body. I do not mind the little protruding belly when I breathe in deeply and fill it with air. In fact, I am feeling like a happy little Buddha. And when I exhale deeply I feel my belly muscles massaging my gut. Focused breathing helps me to be more aware of myself and my surroundings and exercises my abdominal and chest muscles. Talk about sitting down and keeping fit!

Of course, we cannot underestimate the "mind." The mind is brilliant and worth the spotlight it draws! Without the mind and the opposable thumb we would still be beating each other with rocks. However, sometimes when the mind is running overtime it disrupts our parasympathetic nervous system, which is responsible for relaxing and renewing the body, and the result is stress and poor digestion and bowel movements. Yikes! The mind is like a busy monkey, constantly active, full of tricks, craving attention. My personal monkey is a shape shifter and a cunning psychologist – kind of like a Marvel Comics villain. I remember when I was taking a monthlong massage training at the Esalen Institute in Big Sur, California. My instructors, Oliver Bailey and Char Pias, started every morning class with a short meditation. For me, meditation was the hardest part of the training.

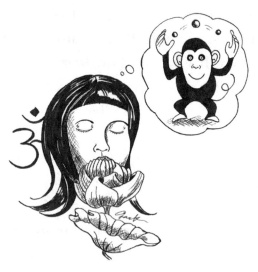

In a class of twenty-six people, we would sit cross-legged in a circle. The palm-size copper Tibetan meditation bowl would sing in G note when Oliver would ring it to mark the beginning of the meditation practice. I would be fidgeting to find a comfortable position, trying to be present, but my mind would be thinking about the past and contemplating the future. Then I would think about the people I liked and didn't like, while at the same time judging myself. My mind was so busy focusing on *everything* that I missed the whole point of "quieting my mind." It was like playing a game of "Shut Up."

"Shshsh, I am meditating here would you please be quiet?" I pleaded with myself.

"No, that's just what I do. If I don't think how can you be certain you exist?"

"Oh, shut up!"

"No, you shut up!"

"Would you shut up about the shut-ups?"

"No! Remember, without me you are not even materialized."

You see what I meant by my mind being like a villain? I was so worried about not doing a good job on meditation until Oliver said, "It's OK to let whatever comes to your mind come in. Don't judge it. Let it be. Recognize it and move on."

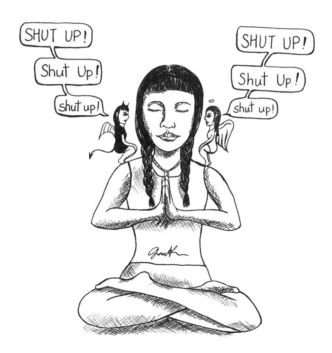

OK. I would recognize my villain and let her pass. My villain showed me many terrifying images with doubts, fears, even death. And from somewhere within me another source of strength, faith and beauty emerged. The feeling was of refreshing, cooling spring water rushing through my veins. The connection with my body extended to the trees outside the window, the earth, the sky, and back into me. I then became the trees, the earth, and the sky. I was infinitely tiny and gigantic at the same time. The micro- and macrocosmic were one. And then everything started to fade. I was just floating in space, but I was not afraid. A sense of peace and calm wrapped around me. Like a baby in a warm blanket, I felt safe and happy. This sense of happiness is now within me and I retrieve it whenever I want to.

In my massage practice now, before a client shows up I clear my own receptor field, letting go of judgments of myself and others, feelings of doubt, attachment to the outcome of the massage session. I go in with an open mind and heart. I go in knowing that each of my clients is also my teacher. They all teach me different ways to work with the body, how to listen to their body, and most of all how to take their feedback not as criticism but as a tool to improve for the next session. Each massage session is an opportunity for me to practice my self-awareness and awareness of others. Massage is meditation.

When I am focused and grounded in my own body I can provide undivided attention to my clients. During a massage session I invite my clients to sink into their body by using audible breathing. Often their breathing pattern will sync up with mine. With some super-duper cerebral clients, I give them little instructions to follow.

"Let's take a deep breath in and take a deep breath out. Feel the rise and fall of your belly. Follow with your chest and then your shoulders. One more time. Inhale through your nose and exhale through your mouth. On your next exhalation, let your body completely melt into the massage table. Feel my hands resting on your shoulders and moving down your back when you exhale. Breathe into the area where my hands are resting or moving."

If the mind is too active to be turned off during a massage session, at least it can focus on the minute changes going on within the body. Another tool I like to use is taking my client on an imaginary tour. I use this technique when none of my fancy manual massage techniques has worked and I feel a strong resistance from my client.

"Now imagine you are sitting on a beach," I say. "The sand is soft, you are digging your toes in, wiggling them around because it feels so good to have the sand move between them. You feel the warm sand on your legs, hips and everywhere the sand touches you. You feel a sense of comfort. You can relax and let go of any tension you are holding onto. You dig your hands in the sand and pretend you are playing piano keys. This tingling feeling extends all the way from your fingertips to your hands, forearms and shoulders. Your back, neck and head are extending and elongating with ease. They move freely with every twist and turn. The ocean breeze is soothing, touching every inch of your skin, opening your pores. You feel your skin breathing in life-giving energy and ridding your being of foul stagnation. The wave of the ocean is talking to your internal organs. The rhythm of the ebb and flow is aligning your internal and external body. Your body and mind are one. You are one."

BODY + MIND = 1

The mind-body connection is a beautiful thing to behold. A sigh, a twitch – these are ways the body can release tension and drift off to a peaceful place, not asleep but deep at rest. Upledger CranioSacral Therapy, founded by Dr. John E. Upledger, an osteopathic physician, calls the state a "Still Point," and in stillness the body has the chance to focus on repair and rejuvenation. The slow, still and sometimes soft touch is contrary to what we are exposed to every day. Our cardiovascular, circulatory, digestive, endocrine, integumentary, immune, lymphatic, musculoskeletal, nervous, respiratory, reproductive and urinary systems all get a chance to breathe. Ah, how nice it is just to breathe, and just be.

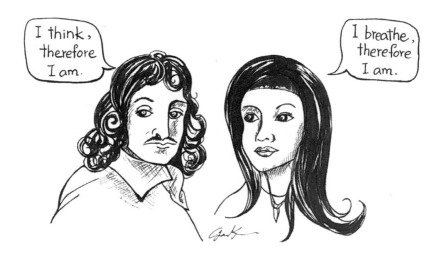

In the massage setting with your partner, the practice of being present can be the most challenging, but it is vitally important. With my husband, I tend to chatter on about what happened to me at work or nag him about dirty dishes, bills that need to be paid, or the mac and cheese our daughter did not eat. It is as if I leave the serene, calm, centered person at work and assume a different identity once I get back home. I was not being present nor nurturing to him, and in fact, it was quite the opposite: I was being really annoying and it was all about "me."

In his book *Nonviolent Communication* Marshall B. Rosenberg talks about how empathy is to empty our mind and listen with our whole being. He introduces Chinese philosopher Chuang-Tzu's insight on this subject:

"The hearing that is only in the ear is one thing. The hearing of the understanding is another. But the hearing of the spirit is not limited to any one faculty, to the ear, or to the mind. Hence it demands the emptiness of all the faculties. And when the faculties are empty, then the whole being listens. There is then a direct grasp of what is right there before you that can never be heard with the ear or understood with the mind."

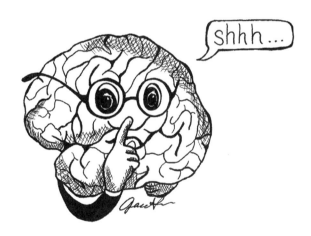

Rosenberg also reminds us that true empathy means before we quickly give advice, reassure, or express our own feelings, we ask the listener if that is indeed what he or she is needing. Empathy for others and ourselves fosters the space we all need to be in the present. That is right: empathy for ourselves too. In my own scenario, after working all day, commuting an hour back home, I ask to have forty minutes to myself to have a snack, take a walk in the woods, and take a shower before I can continue being the nurturer. I need to take care of my own needs or else I find myself turning into a low blood-sugar were-wolf. So, consider yourself warned.

Being present and creating a nurturing space for your partner is so healing that you will find your mutual connection naturally deepening. Some of the best massage I have ever received was from my husband, who has less than no official massage training. He was focused and present with his touch. When you are present, you open up space for healing, which extends to your partner through intention. Listen with your hands: *Is the body asking for gentle, nurturing touch? Is the body yearning for focused pressure points? Or does the body want deep work? Or maybe a combination of all of them?* Trust your hands and let them guide you.

3

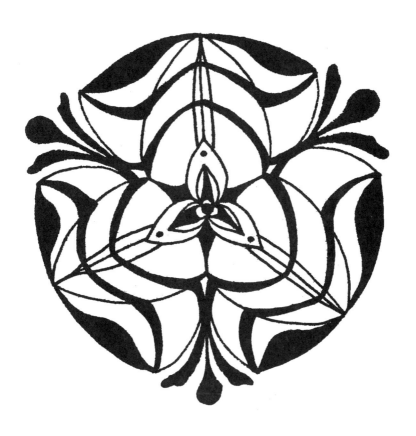

'Your massage is better than sex!'
~ Maggie~

I love sexy rubs. The candles, soft music, lavender-scented lotion, soft sheets, plush blanket – it's all great. And with any kind of luck that will all lead to passionate sex. Of course, if you have children, you know that first you have to feed them, give them a bath, put them to bed and read two bedtime stories. Then you quickly get yourself cleaned up and maybe slip into that semi-see-through nightgown and that uncomfortable tiny G-string, leaving you, oh, maybe an hour before both you and your partner are too tired to do anything. Sounds exhausting. Foreplay might be the only thing on the menu tonight. Or skip foreplay all together and just get down and get dirty. And the next day skip the ambience and sexy rubs. And within a couple of years, sex becomes something that you occasionally do when it is convenient.

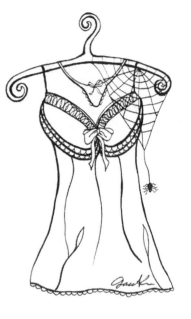

Esther Perel did a TED Talk on "the secret to desire in a long-term relationship." One of the most interesting concepts she shared was that "foreplay is not something we do before sex but is the time after sex and before the next one begins." Massage is the ultimate foreplay for you and your partner. Massage is sustainable, continuous bliss for the giver and the receiver. Loving, nurturing, caring touch deepens the connection with the one you love. And the best part? You already know how to do it. It is an innate human behavior. We only forget because we are out of practice. Practice by being present. Be the one who really listens and hears what your partner says and also understands his or her body language. Be present and one with him or her. Not thinking about work promotion, dirty dishes and laundry, setting up play dates for the kids, what to cook for dinner, calling back and making up an excuse why you have not called your mother, questioning the extra charge on the phone bill, or how the guest toilet really needs a good scrubbing. You are in the same time and space with your partner, not in the past or the future but right here, right now. Yes, it sounds good on paper. You are nodding as you read these words in front of you. But in reality it takes conscious effort to be in the now.

i am that pebble
i am that twig
i am that cliff
i am that water
i close my eyes
breathing in the moment
i open my eyes
expect scenes to change
everything seems to remain
except my mind
wandering from point to point
the wave flows in and out
things come in focus
and go out in blur
what is constant?
when i do not remain the same
do i find comfort in the constant
do i find inspiration in the ever changing
i am that duality

i am the morning glory
the sunrise
the breeze
the spider
the good
the bad
the ugly
today i am the mistress of my thoughts
i am the blessed angel
who is soaking up the sun ray
i am the laughing child
who is dancing under the stars
i am the pretty maiden
who is bathing in the moonlight
i weep for all the gratitude i have
i am the humble human knowing
mortality will catch up with me someday
i pretend i have all the tomorrows
i lay down my guards
i put things off for another day
i dwell in the past
i am the humble human who
is blessed angel
is getting lost in the
what-ifs, should-ofs, could-ofs and would-ofs
i step back looking at me from the outside
how funny the human drama
the tense jaws, tight fists, raised eyebrows, shallow breath
all for what?
the perception of some kind of reality?
i look at the world through the same eyes

but a softer gaze
i breathe in the world through the same lungs
but with more gratitude
i feel the world through the same heart
but with more acceptance
i am that i am

There is an illusion that we have to be constantly planning for what's happening next. We create lists of to-dos in our minds, on our smart phones, computers, Post-It notes, whiteboards and calendars. We think we need to think or we cease to exist. Take a moment once in a while just to *be*. I live in the Santa Cruz Mountains with my family, and every Sunday my daughter, Eureka, and I roll the trash can down to Highway 9 for Monday morning pick-up. One Sunday just like every other Sunday, we slowly walked down the hill while I pushed the can with one hand and held Eureka's hand with another. Like most grown-ups my head was full of things that needed to be done, and all of a sudden Eureka let go of my hand and ran in front of me.

She stretched out her little hand with authority in front of me and yelled, "Stop!"

Then she said, "Mommy do this."

She kneeled down, hands in prayer position and said "Namaste" to the redwood trees.

She asked me to do the same. At first, I felt silly, but once I stopped and took the time to observe everything that was around me, I realized how blessed I am to be her mother and to be surrounded by fresh air, wild flowers and giant trees. I laughed with joy. My three-year-old taught me a great lesson on being in the moment. The present of the present is now the essence.

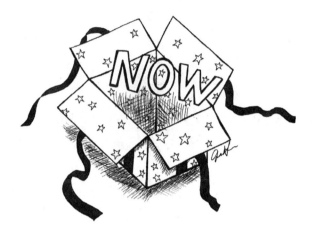

Feel the air warming up in your nose and traveling from your nose and spreading out to the branches of your lungs. The diaphragm rises, filling every organ and blood vessel with life-giving oxygen. Feel the expansion of every cell and sense, and slowly exhale. The body relaxes. Any tension that is stored in the face – between the brows, around the eyes, in the jaw line – is starting to let go. The muscles in the front and back of the neck lengthen, creating more space for the shoulders and the colarbones to rest. The arms, elbows, wrists and fingers lengthen as if there is an invisible light source shooting out from each fingertip. The sternum, shoulder blades, front and back of the rib cages, and belly muscles come closer together and squeeze out any remaining carbon dioxide and massage the internal organs. The hips, knees, ankles and toes are free of movement. Cervical, thoracic, lumbar, sacral – about all of the thirty-three of the spinal vertebrae are filled with nourishing cerebrospinal fluid that travels from the cranium to the tailbone and back to the cranium. The cranial sutures, joints, tendons, ligaments, muscles and blood vessels expand and contract with the rhythm of the universe. Inhalation and exhalation.

Feel the sensation of the cloth you are wearing touching your skin. Feel the socks on your feet and inside the shoes. What's the texture? Does the sensation change with inhalation and exhalation? If you are sitting, notice which part of your butt is touching the chair. Is it toward the back, where you can feel your tailbone? Or is it toward the middle where you are actually sitting on your sit bones? Maybe it's more toward the front where you are hunching over? If you are standing, is your weight on the heels or balls of your feet? Are you putting more weight on one foot? Are your knees slightly bent or are they locked rigidly? Are you sucking in your gut? Are you breathing fully? Are your shoulders relaxed or are they raised? Are they pulled toward your chest, pulled way back, or happily resting at your side? Is your neck extended forward? Is it more comfortable to turn to one side than the other? How are you feeling in your body now?

Shake out your hands, wrists, elbows and shoulders. Now move your neck from side to side, front to back, make circles, clockwise and counterclockwise, and do the same movement with your hips. Now without moving your upper body, move your hips only. Put your hands on your knees and make tiny circles both to the right and left and feel your ankles moving along with the knees. Jump up and down. Do a somersault. Wave your arms. Kick your legs. Make funny faces if you like. Shake out your whole body and make whatever sound you wish. Yell out, sing out, or whisper. Get rid of any excess energy and get the stagnant parts moving.

During the birth of this book several Google massage

therapists and I were in Jean Couch's Body Mechanic work-shop co-taught by Jenn Sherer from the company Spinefulness at the Balance Centre in Palo Alto. Man, was I out of balance, even with the stringent Catholic upbringing! Who would have guessed that?! I have always been told that I had good posture, but apparently I had an over-corrected one, which meant I sucked my gut in and puffed my chest out like Foghorn Leg-horn. My gut was sucked in because I was too self-conscious. This made it difficult for me to breathe fully. Can you imagine walking around with half-breath most of the time? I silently recited to myself, "The corset days are over and the happy Bud-dha days are in." The puffed-up chest caused my back to con-tract, which created tension between the vertebrae. The mystery of my backache was solved! To help eliminate and prevent back pain, Jean and Jenn reminded me to stand with my toes pointing out diagonally, knees slightly bent, and with my weight on my heels so that when I looked down I could see my ankles. It felt awkward because my proprioception was telling me my butt was sticking out too far, but in truth it was not. When it came to correct sitting, I was reminded to sit on my sit bone, relax my

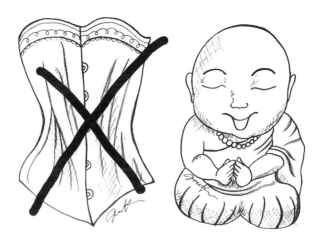

quads by lowering the knees, and relax my ribcage. Wow, it was really challenging, but I knew if I kept on with the practice my body would eventually remember what to do. Another important correction was to bring my chin back so my neck wasn't overextended. Do you know the weight of the head will increase by ten pounds with every inch it leans forward? I learned that in the class and was astonished! It took me a couple of seconds to realize what I was hearing. "Really? That's crazy!" No wonder tension in the upper back, neck and shoulders is so common. These great teachers also reminded me to bring my shoulders back so they were comfortably situated by my sides, not rolled forward

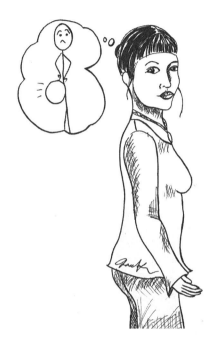

or backward. To unlearn and relearn standing and sitting is an ongoing process for me. I check my spine to determine if a particular vertebra needs to be adjusted by either moving my spine forward or backward, and I practice that every day. So if you see me moving my hands up and down on my back, or touching my chin, or checking my pelvis and looking down at my ankles, it is not because I have an itch or am trying to avoid eye contact. Honestly!

Slowly come to a still point. Feel your feet rooted on the ground and extended to the center of the earth. Your arms gently rest at your sides. Breathe in and draw up the earth energy from your feet to your legs and hips. The spinal discs

34

are stacking one by one on top of each other with space and fluids for ease of movement. Your head is resting effortlessly on top of the cervical spine. It feels like there is a string connected to the top of your head, pulling you toward the sky. Draw the heaven energy to your crown, which is charging with positive energy. Breathe out and recycle all the energy back into the earth through your feet. Remember the body is three-dimensional:Feel the relationship of your body with your surroundings.

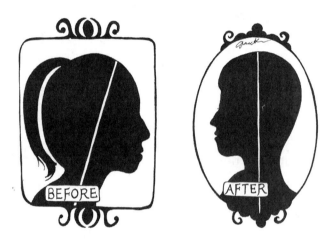

Feel the air element that is moving through you and wrapping around you. Feel the earth element you are standing on that is holding you. Feel the water element you are made of and that is flowing through you. Feel the fire element that is living beneath the ground and within your body. You are made of star dust. Every element that is in the universe is within you.

Stand with your feet about shoulder-width apart, knees slightly bent, hips aligned with shoulders. Breathe deeply into your belly, push your belly button as far away from you as possible, and breathe out by drawing your belly button as close to your spine as possible. Rub your hands together and feel the heat forming in your palms. Slowly pull your palms away and bring them closer together while keeping the sensation of heat between them. Repeat this movement several times and see how far your hands can be apart while still feeling the heat. Some people describe the sensation forming between the palms as tingling, sticky or magnetic. What you are feeling right now, my friend, is *energy*. What is energy? And how can you prove it is in your hands? Is it real or is it imaginary? And what if I cannot feel anything? Am I totally hopeless?

Before I answer these questions, I would like to share a story from Dr. John Upledger. In his book *Your Inner Physician and You*, he talks about healing energy: "What is it? I don't know. I do know when it works, it moves the instruments that we use to measure electricity. I know that, when it works, the previously mentioned heat release occurs and the previously described 'therapeutic pulse' crescendos and decrescendos. I know that during the time that it is working the craniosacral system comes to a standstill. What is it? I don't know, but it works."

Energy is everywhere. It is around you, it is in you. You are an energetic being. Your body transforms the food you consume into usable energy. When you rub your hands together you are creating motion and kinetic energy. Heat is the evidence of energy. What you are feeling between your palms is real energy, not imaginary. And if you cannot feel anything, that does not mean energy does not exist. It means you have more noticing to do – noticing the heat that is created by rubbing your hands together, that the center of your palm is warmer than your fingertips perhaps, that your hands are dry or a little sweaty. Just noticing. Energy follows intention. By focusing your intention that is gathering energy in your hands you are indeed gather-

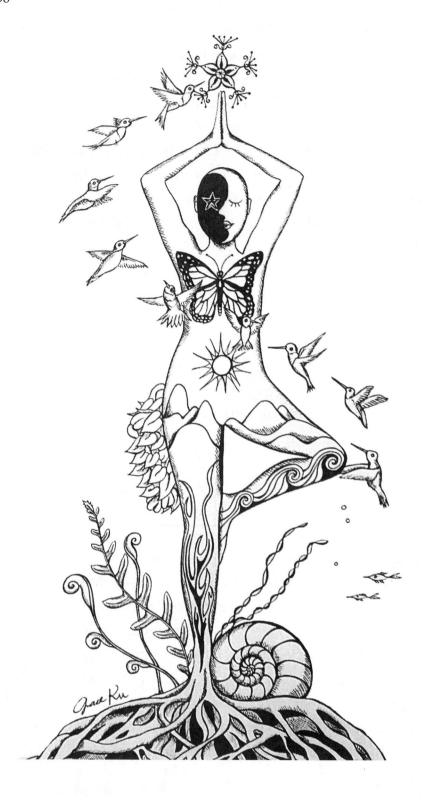

ing energy from within yourself and the universe. Energy is traveling from the universe to you to the earth and back to the universe. It is moving in a continuous, circular motion. Albert Einstein: "Energy cannot be created or destroyed, it can only be changed from one form to another." So you see, by being present and focusing your intention you are able to "move" energy.

Over a weekend at the Esalen Institute at Big Sur, I had the wonderful opportunity to study Spiritual Massage with Maria Lucia Bittencourt Sauer and her assistant Bo. Bo had been living with the Hopi tribe in Arizona and learning their shamanic ways. We started the class by burning sage to cleanse the space and ourselves, then followed with a shamanic journey, led by Bo, to find our power animals. With the sound of his drum, my mind's eye saw a redwood forest; as I was walking, the scenery changed to a path that led me to a waterfall, then a tunnel appeared and I went in with the intention of looking for my spirit animal. A deer appeared. I told myself, "Oh, no, not a deer! It's too predictable and she is too weak. I want something that is stronger." Just as I was thinking, a rabbit showed himself to me. "No, no, not a rabbit! Rabbits are too sweet, not tough enough. I want a powerful animal." Not an eagle, a wolf nor a bear showed up. Instead, there was a tiny robin waiting for me at the other end of the tunnel. I shared my journey with the class and tried not to sound disappointed. Bo said, "Deer medicine is a strong medicine, she is compassionate and gentle. When she comes to you, that means you have something to learn. Even ant medicine is powerful." I learned my lesson to be open without the need to judge.

Maria shared her techniques combining Brazilian and Chinese approaches to energy work, ranging from grounding with earthly energy to receiving heavenly energy. She showed us how to get rid of static energy, including past aches, pains and hurtful things that our body still holds on to. She said, "Let go of all the old patterns that we are holding on to and make our body lighter, so we can expand and grow. Invite your spirit to come and occupy your wonderful body – fully." Energetic work does not require physical contact with the receiver; in this particular workshop we touched the physical body half the time. Even during the time we were in direct contact with the body our focus was on the spiritual body. My partner Akiko had a profound release during both hands-on and hands-off technique. Maria reminded us that we need to be mindful of our thoughts because everything is created internally, then manifests itself outwardly. As a receiver I fell fast asleep, my hands twitched from time to time, and that was all I could remember. Upon awakening I felt a sense of peace and gratitude.

On the second day we journeyed again with the shamanic drumming. I entered another cave much like the Waitomo Cave in New Zealand, full of glowworms, but instead of stalactites it was hanging with clear crystals. I was not a bit surprised when the deer appeared again. This time she had antlers that looked like trees. She looked ancient, wise and magical. Then she told me she was not just a deer, she was an Elemental spirit. She asked me to join her, and together we bent down and drank the spring water. At that precise moment I became her, she was me, we were one. The water was clear, the cave echoed with the water drops, the glowworms' light reflected from the crystal, all so foreign and yet familiar. We explored the cave, and what a beautiful sight to behold! We gathered the courage to explore outside the cave, knowing that the outside world might not be safe. Once we were out, we felt the soft sunlight on our skin and the green grass rolling under our feet and brushing against our legs. Then a Bengal tiger strolled majestically into view, a brownish rat playfully made his appearance, and we saw a white owl watching us from a treetop. I came back from the journey feeling connected with life. When I shared my journey with the class we found out the tiger was Maria's spiritual animal and the rat and the owl were spiritual animals of other classmates. Somehow we all met in this dreamlike world. Coincidence?

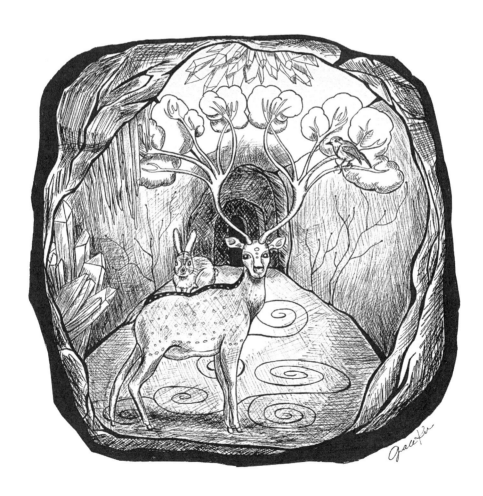

During one massage session at Google I applied acupressure for an engineer who was going through some life changes. His body was open to receive the work and he felt calm and peaceful afterward. However, he was having a hard time wrapping his mind around what had just happened. He suggested we conduct an experiment to prove the existence of energy and establish that what he felt was real.

We walked to Charleston Park, next to Google's main campus, and from a plastic bag he pulled out an oven mitt and a sheet of baking foil. I brought along a palm-sized, clear crystal ball and a rose quartz. We sat facing each other on a wooden bench, among well-manicured, blossoming cherry trees and tall snake grass. A manmade waterfall gurgled nearby. With eyes closed we rubbed our hands together to create heat in our palms, then gradually pulled our hands apart while maintaining the unseen connection. The engineer opened his eyes with a look of amazement. The connection between our palms was warm, sticky, round, elastic, fluid and infinite. He then put the oven mitt on his right hand and we went back to concentrating on the sensation in our hands. Was there any difference? For those of you holding your breath, the answer is: No. Nada. The oven mitt did not disturb the energy flow at all.

Next up: the foil. My client fashioned makeshift mittens out of the foil for each of his hands and we tried again. Facing him and seeing him with foil hands, it was hard for me not to bust out laughing. The foil made the energy feel "cooler," but that was it. OK, now it was my turn to bring out the crystal and quartz. I had them in my hands during this final trial. The concentration of energy work heated up the rocks fast and the weight in my hands made me feel more grounded, but I was not able to detect a quality change within the energy itself. In this one-hour experiment my client concluded that energy does exist and can be raised when we concentrate and direct our attention, in this case to our hands. For me it was great to witness how energy follows intention and that anyone can learn to cultivate it!

My personal experience on intention and touch dates back to preschool. When I fell and got ouches at home, my mom would blow air on the scratches, clean up the wound, and put on a bandage. She would kiss it and gently pat my head and tell me everything would be fine. Her voice, the look in her eyes, and her care made a whole world of difference to me. When I fell in school, one of the teachers would clean up the wound and also put on a bandage, but I would still feel hurt. Part of me knew the mechanical part of me was taken care of but somehow something was missing.

In my professional practice and personal life, I imagine my clients and my partner as children who need more than just a mechanical rub. I give them my full attention and compassion without judgment: feeling honored by their openness to receive, feeling elated to witness positive change, feeling blessed for their trust. Setting intention for a positive outcome for your partner, being present, gathering your energy, following your partner's breath and trusting your intuition are the most important skills, tools and mediation for giving a great massage. You might call them the ultimate foreplay, lasting anywhere from fifteen minutes or less to two hours or more. So let's get started!

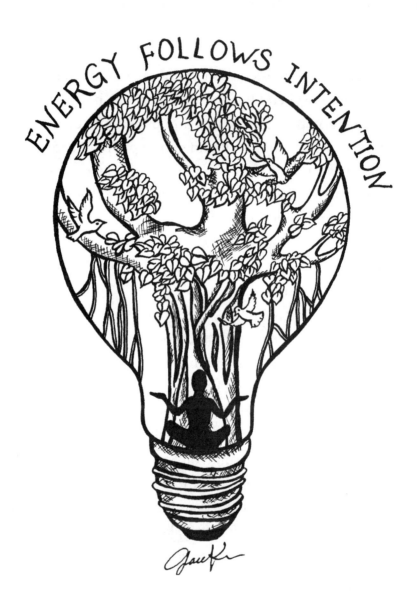

4

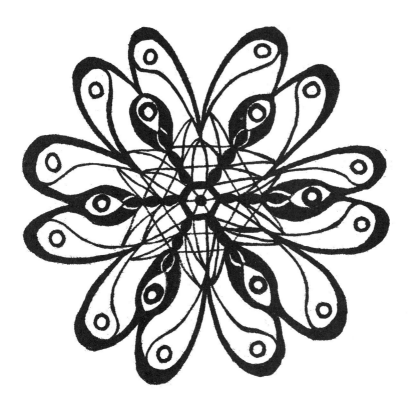

Don't go to bed angry – or without a massage!

"Not tonight, I'm tired." Sound familiar? I know I say that at least a couple of times a month. These are words that leave one person feeling rejected and another feeling guilty, but learning to do great massage with your partner can help avoid them – and great massage does not need to be an exhausting, back-breaking experience. To the contrary, with the right approach it can be relaxing, reviving and rejuvenating. Begin by making whatever time you have with your partner a sacred ceremony, a time to look into each other's eyes and honor your connection. Again, it doesn't have to be long (though it can be): Ten deeply meaningful minutes together will last a lifetime. Create a space that is safe from the hurry and worry of daily life. Leave mundane burdens behind when you enter your sacred space. This is a giant bubble of happiness where you are accepted just the way you are. Even your most vulnerable, uninhibited self is welcome to relax, surrender and let go. You are perfect the way you are because you are the god and goddess of your domain. So it's OK to let down your guard and be in the moment and, as Joseph Campbell put it, "Follow your bliss." This is where the magic begins.

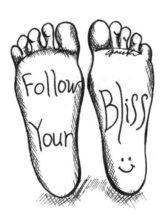

First Magic: Enchanting Moments, for when you have only fifteen minutes or less. Ask your partner which areas of her body most crave attention – with limited time, it's better to focus on one or two areas rather than rush to cover the whole body. A hurried massage will feel like a freight train running over her. If she can't pinpoint a zone, that's OK; make it into a game. Write down different parts of the body on separate pieces of paper, fold them up, and have her pick a couple. You can also blindfold her, increasing the excitement of the unexpected and putting her focus on your touch.

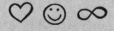

Trick of the Trade

Blindfold
Having the eyes covered while receiving massage heightens the sensation of touch and helps the receiver to be more grounded in her body. It's particularly useful for someone who spends a lot of time in her head and has a hard time letting go.

One day at Google I had a client who had signed up for a

half-hour massage. He came running in straight from a meeting, ten minutes late for his appointment and frazzled. I asked him which area of his body he wanted me to focus on.

He quickly said, "Neck, shoulder, back and legs. And I like deep pressure"

I paused before answering and looked at him steadily.

"Realistically, with the time we have today we can do more good focusing on one or two areas," I said. "And we will go as deep as your body allows. Do you have one area that really stands out to you right now?"

We focused on his back with the time we had and saw great improvement afterward. He left feeling more relaxed and happy. Later, he sent me an email to let me know he had booked another session in two weeks. All because some simple communication had helped us set realistic expectations that could be fulfilled.

I didn't always have the confidence to be so forthright. In the very beginning of my massage career I often worried about whether my clients would like my technique or even me as a person, so I tried too hard to please them. Back then I would have said yes to a crazy neck-shoulder-back-legs-deep-pressure request and powered through the entire body in less than a half-hour, thinking I was doing a good job. I would go as deep as humanly possible, even if it meant I might hurt myself. I did not have the courage to communicate truthfully and I took every suggestion personally.

I remember meeting this one particular female client while working in a boutique spa in San Mateo. She was very exacting – she demanded deep tissue work on her back, and I could only use my fingertips. For me the session was an hour of excruciating pain. She couldn't relax and I was uncomfortable working with her. She kept telling me how she used to see this male massage therapist, clearly trying to get me to duplicate his massage moves. It was a total disaster. I could never be like her ex-therapist! If I had the courage to tell her, this is what I should have said: "First, I am not your ex-therapist, so please do not expect to have the same massage. Second, using only fingertips to work is not safe for me. I need to alternate my tools, using my fist, forearm and elbow, and I will be very attentive to your needs in doing so. Third, if you find today's session does not address your needs, please try another therapist." It's a good thing I outgrew the insecurity that prevented me from forthright communication, or I might have given up massage a long time ago.

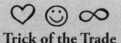

Trick of the Trade

Massage Pressure

There seems to be a myth out there that if a massage does not hurt it is not working. An effective massage does not need to be hurtful! To the contrary, some of the most effective massage techniques, such as craniosacral therapy, only require five grams of pressure.

If the pressure is too great, the muscles tighten up and the massage turns into a tough-man contest. Save your hands by having your partner's body work

48

ing with you instead of against you. Take time to
warm up the muscle before going deeper, and only
increase the pressure if the body allows you to. So be
patient: Wait until the body tells you to go, then you
move on.

Second Magic: Bewitching Spell, for the rare occasion
when all the stars are aligned and you, the lucky angel, get to
spend an hour or more lavishing undivided attention on your
partner. I believe giving a full body massage is in your cards.
Light up the candles, bring out the scented massage lotion, put
on music you can both relax into, and, most importantly, keep
your partner warm. A key to giving a relaxing full-body massage is to use as little draping as possible, allowing you to dance
your fingers, palms, forearms, elbows on your partner's body
without having to stop, uncover the draping, stop, and cover
him back up again. A fluid dance calms the mind and soothes
the nerve. Remember, good massage isn't about putting on
blinders and proceeding to do your own thing; you need to be
ultra-aware of your partner's responses. Tune in to his rhythm
of breath and movement of body, and watch for any significant
shifts – and the insignificant ones too. Observe how his body
reacts when you slow down or change the pressure.

Esalen-style massage is well known for its fluid, graceful
and nurturing touch. Newcomers to massage often work sys-
tematically, seeing the body as quadrants made up of different

parts; Esalen is less formulaic. The body is one being. Esalen massage is inspired by the ocean wave, the continuous movement down along the body from the top of the head to the tips of the toes and back up again. From the head moving down to the arm, moving up from the arm and going down the glutes, down the leg. Moving up from the leg, to the back, and to the other arm. There is no specific place where you should start or end the massage. The only "rule" is that you maintain a continuous connection your moves feel more complete when you begin the next move where you ended earlier. Again, you are dancing with the body, and how you choreograph your dance is up to you and your partner.

   The month I was training at the Esalen Institute, I was surprised by how a simple effleurage could be so powerful. The class practiced that single massage move – with your partner lying face down in the "prone position," the long stroke gliding from the base of the neck, to the sacrum, and back to the neck – for an hour. There were so many subtle changes of pressure within that one move that I had never taken the time to explore or notice. For example, the pressure is light when the hands are on the base of the neck, increases when reaching the mid scapular, decreases once you are close to the last rib, and increases on the sacrum with a push toward the tailbone. From there: Parting the hands on top of the glutes, wrap your fingers around the hip bone, pulling it toward your partner's head, and bring your hands up to the mid scapulas, pushing the scapulas apart. Slowly move the hands to the top of the shoulders and, pushing down toward your partner's feet, bring the hands to the base of the neck. My partner, Kaiko, was out cold on the table within the first three minutes of practice. I looked around and saw more classmates were falling asleep. Michael started his famous snoring sonata, which echoed throughout the wooden yurt. Soon, snoring in other keys and tempos joined in to create a sleepy symphony. I tried not to laugh, but it was hard. Effleurage can be extended to the whole body once you are comfortable exploring. We will discuss more technique in section two -- Ingredients.

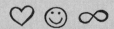

Trick of the Trade

Massage Lotion
Unscented massage lotion is a good choice for beginners because it has more "grip," providing traction when deeper pressure is needed. I find lotion also works better on people who have more body hair. You can use essential oil to add aromatherapy to your session. It is said that our sense of smell is the strongest link to our subconscious, with highly sensitive olfactory nerves, olfactory bulbs and nerve endings sending messages directly to the brain. Before using any essential oil, be sure you and your partner do not have skin sensitivity issues.

Third Magic: Hypnotic Tonic. Scalp, face, neck, shoulder, hands and feet are sort of the foolproof recipe for an intimate encounter without having to undress. You can do this in a public space with no fear of getting arrested or setting a bad example for innocent children. I see it a lot: Parents get uncomfortable with other couples' public displays of affection, grow flustered and embarrassed, and quickly get their children and pull them away. Or some people whistle and yell, "Oh, get a room!" I just chuckle at these reactions. As my friend Eric said during one massage session, "At some point we all have to realize that we have a body." The body loves and adores to be loved and adored! Be embarrassed about not tipping your waitress, or pretending you didn't see your door ding the other car, or lying about some of your habits, but don't ever be embarrassed about showing your partner how much you care by massaging her in public. Well, maybe massaging her feet in a restaurant might be a little unsanitary. Otherwise, it's all good.

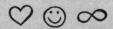

Trick of the Trade

Helping Your Partner to Relax
When your partner has a hard time relaxing, gently tap on a tight muscle and do an audible breathing. The tapping serves as a cue for the body to know exactly which muscle is tensing up, and the audible breathing reminds the body to relax.

The neck and shoulders appreciate gentle, rhythmic squeeing, strong focused pressure, supported rotation and traction as well as energetic work. An average adult-size head weighs about ten pounds – that is close to the weight of a big newborn baby. Imagine being the neck, carrying and supporting this big baby more than sixteen hours a day. A pain in the neck is very common, so simply placing one hand on his forehead and squeezing his neck muscles with another can provide a great relief. And of course there are the shoulders that are connected to the neck. The neck and shoulders are like fraternal twins, they obviously do not look alike and yet they share this mysterious bond in which one reflects anothers' feelings. After

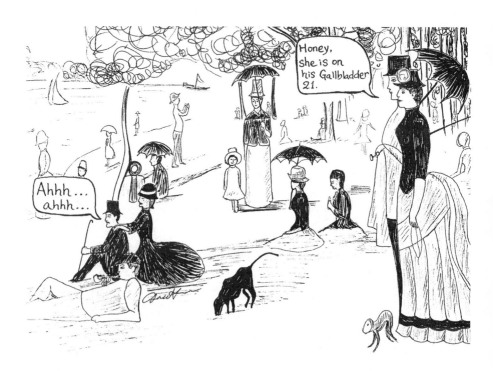

taking care of the neck let us give a little love to his shoulder. The trapezius connects the neck and shoulder and is shaped like a mini superman's cape. This cape gets tangled and needs straightening more often than we realize. To untangle this article of clothing, first squeeze, second stretch, third repeat the first and second steps till you see the desired result. It is also refreshing to apply acupressure technique on the shoulder. For example, Gallbladder 21, in the middle top of the shoulder, facilitates shoulder tension release. You could be sitting in the park, gazing out into the sunset while working on his Gallbladder 21, right out of a Georges Seurat painting.

The scalp, face, hands and feet have more nerve endings than the back, so very little goes a long way, although some people really like deep work on the scalp and feet. Believe it or not, controlled hair pulling can be extremely rejuvenating and relaxing at the same time. My first time receiving it, I wasn't sure if it was pain or pleasure. It seems my sensory response was blurred between the two.

The feet carry our weight and often suffer the abuse of shoes that aren't necessarily designed for ease of walking. Yes, we women sometimes have a weakness for shoes that look great with our outfits. I would wager some men secretly do, as well. Comfy, feet-friendly sneakers might be best for our feet, but with a sexy little black dress that's a fashion faux pas.

All the little piggies deserve equal attention, whether it's the one that went to market, stayed home, had roast beef, had none, or went "Wee wee wee" all the way home. Reflexology charts map out the corelations between points on the soles and different places on the body. It might look like a foot massage, but you could be massaging your partner's heart while reading her love poems.

Trick of the Trade

Creating Your Own Self-Massage Device
Now let us explore some fun ways to take care of our body by incorporating everyday objects, a la MacGyver (although I have yet to try duct tape or paper clips). One day after working with four clients, I felt a kink in my neck, and my forearms were pretty sore too. I went down to the Google cafe and picked up a bottle of cold water and a hot burrito. I placed the burrito on my neck and rolled the cold bottle on my forearms. The heat from the burrito was a welcome sensation on my neck, and the cold on my forearms helped to soothe the tired muscles. I then used cross-fiber technique to work on the forearms, followed by stretching. I laced my fingers together behind my head, leaned back, and my thumbs went naturally into the base of my skull. After holding that spot for half a minute or so, I moved my thumbs farther apart along the base of my skull, then stretched. The burrito had already relaxed my neck, the thumbs were guiding my focus, and by breathing deeply into those areas the knot had my undivided attention. Not to mention, I got a nice burrito and water for a snack.

Tennis balls come in handy when you want to get at that tight spot on your back. Tape two of them together (hey, we just found a good use for the duct tape!), squat down in front of a wall, then lean back with your homemade massager pressed horizontally against the upper back. Slowly stand up, allowing your high-tech device to roll down your back. Voila! Adjust the pressure by modifying the force you apply against the balls. Simple to operate and small enough to take it anywhere….One tennis ball is all you need to massage the sole of your foot. Stand up and push your foot into the ball. Let it roll around a bit – it is surprisingly comfortable. Play around with balls of different size and density to see what works for your unique build (lacrosse balls, for instance, offer firmer resistance). You see, it is easy to have a ball.

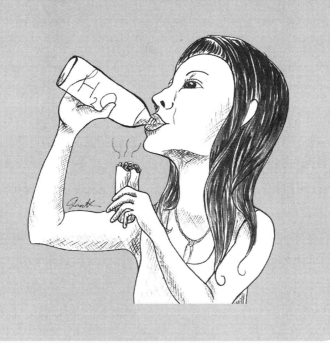

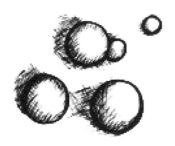

Our hands take their share of abuse throughout the day, as well. Typing on the keyboard, playing sports (and, yeah, carrying a baby and groceries is a sport), lifting weights, gripping a steering wheel intensely, knitting, playing a musical instrument ... you name it, our hands are always contracting and gripping. It can be an amazing relief to your partner when you rotate their wrists, open up the palms, pull on finger joints, unjam the jammed digits. I have had many clients fall asleep while I work on their hands. More than a few have also confessed to me that they find the experience very sensual. Try this: The next time you find yourself getting caught up in a disagreement with your partner, massage her hands. She can't be upset at you while feeling sensual at the same time.

Onward to the face: Did you know there are forty-three muscles in our faces? According to Dr. David Song of the University of Chicago Medical Center, it takes eleven major muscles to frown and twelve major muscles to smile. However, it takes less energy to smile than frown. Our complex facial expressions convey our psyche. "The face you have before thirty is given to you by your parents and after thirty is how you make it." I read that somewhere, and it makes sense. Frowning, the facial muscles are narrowed toward the center and down toward the feet. Smiling, the muscles are widened toward the ears and up toward the top of the head. Simple, right? When you massage your partner remember to make smiley faces for her. One area that is an exception is the temporomandibular joint, commonly know as the TMJ, which gets unexpectedly tight. I sense you are thinking, "Huh?" Try this: place your hands underneath your cheek and clench your teeth. Do you feel the muscles sort of "jumping out"? Follow your fingers to the area where you feel the most change, and then open your mouth as big as possible (it's OK, no one is watching), then close your mouth. The opening and closing of the mouth is made possible by the TMJ. You want to move that down to encourage relaxation of the face. Later in the book, we'll dive deeper into the technique. Craniosacral therapy and acupressure points work beautifully on the face. One gram of pressure to free up the tense facial bones and gentle acupressure points that help to facilitate energy flow are both keys to instant facelifts without a needle or knife.

One afternoon, a new client walked into the spa wanting

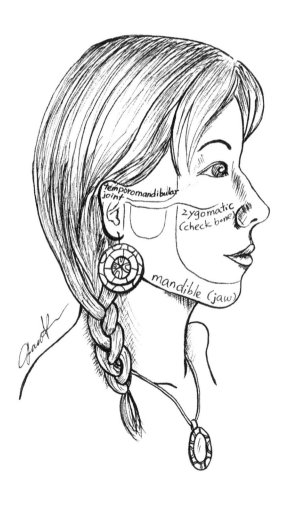

a relaxation massage. He was very quiet and was having a hard time finding a peaceful place. I tried everything I could think of, with no success – until I practiced the art of doing nothing on his face. He let out a huge sigh and started to focus on his breathing. His whole body melted into my hands and onto the massage table. I love the art of doing nothing. It works!

Fourth Magic: Mesmerizing Charms. You know a dog or a cat really likes you when they lie on their back exposing their chest and belly for you to rub. They trust you by showing you their protected, vulnerable side. Same goes with humans. We tend to hold emotional blockages in our chest and abdomen, so when we work with our partner on these areas we need to be extra gentle and kind.

I remember the first time I received acupuncture, back in 2001. I walked into a soft-lit room that smelled of Chinese herb. A beautiful calligraphy piece hung on the wall. Steven Cardoza, my tai chi instructor and also an acupuncturist, checked my pulse, looked at my tongue, and took notes on my family medical history and personal emotional state. As I lay on the table, he put needles in my head, face, chest, arms, legs and, finally, the last one, on the right side of my belly. He asked me to relax and told me he would be back after a bit. I was lying there looking around the room and noticed an embroidered tapestry. I closed my eyes and heard quiet music playing in the background. For whatever reason, I began to cry. An emotional floodgate was opened and sad memories, hurtful feelings, and regretful thoughts tumbled over my seemingly well-composed self. It was uncalled for and I was not prepared to make a scene.

"Wasn't acupuncture supposed to make you feel serene like floating on a cloud? What the fuck?! What is this bullshit?!" I tried to hold back my emotions, but that only amplified the effect. "OK, for whatever unseen wisdom, this needs to happen. So just calm down and be with it." I looked around the treatment room, checking to be sure Steven hadn't returned. I was embarrassed he might see me crying. I lay there and cried god knows for how long. "All right, now the skeleton in my closet is out, hovering over my face with no place to hide. Great, now where is courage when I need it? I am supposed to be the tough one in the family. If I break down now, I don't know what else to be. Fine. I admit I am weak, scared and hurt just like the people I constantly frown upon. I am no better than they are, just better at hiding my personal bullshit. Do I really need to carry this shit around? No. Ha! That's great! I am telling my bullshit to get lost. And it feels absolutely amazing." I came out of that session accepting and loving myself for who I *am*.

We talked a lot about working with the breath. This is no mere buzz phrase among the wellness folks; working with breathing is crucial if you want to provide a nurturing massage for your partner. Expansion, contraction, extension and compression are even more evident when you are on the chest and belly area. Gently rest your hands on your partner, pause and wait until your own breath matches his. Slowly increase the pressure when he exhales and lighten the pressure when he inhales. Try this on yourself first. Place your left hand on your chest and right hand on your belly. Inhale. You'll first notice your belly pushing up your right hand, followed by the movement of your left hand. Exhale and feel your right hand fall first, then your left. Now increase the pressure on both hands when you exhale, putting a little more pressure on the belly. Here comes the fun part: Make a large, clockwise circle with your right hand on the belly while your left hand moves slightly up and down on the chest. Practice this move until you are comfortable, without going eyes crossed and hands twisted.

I remember working as a pre-kindergarten teacher while taking massage class in the evening. One little boy named Derek was having a hard time due to his parents' separation. He did not want to participate in class activity and only wanted to play alone. During nap time he flat-out refused to lie down. So I tried

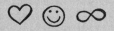

Trick of the Trade

Nurturing Belly Massage
Use the belly button as the center of a spiral. Slowly increase the circle by going clockwise, which comports with the position of the ascending, transverse and descending colon. There are many health articles promoting the benefits of abdominal massage in helping calm colic babies, ease pregnancy tension, and simply for helping regular stressed-out people to relax. Abdominal massage has also proven to help with digestive issues.

massaging his belly, hoping to calm him down. He responded immediately, hugging his Sponge Bob blanket and looking at me with his big eyes. Little by little, I was able to gain his trust, slowly but surely having him take naps with his friends.

Massage is for all of us. Everybody can benefit from loving and caring touch. Remember the famous research done by psychologist Harry Harlow in the 1960s on the nature of affection? He removed baby monkeys from their biological mother six to twelve hours after birth and gave them the choice of two monkey-mommy look-alikes. The first mommy was made of wire and had a baby bottle attached to offer food; the second mommy was made of soft terrycloth, but offered no food. The experiment showed that the baby monkeys spent more time with the soft fake mommy with no food than the wired mommy with food. Seeking and offering affection is innate. The poetry and magic in touch begin with self-awareness, centering and presence, because the real magic is moving from the heart with love. Our hands are extensions of that same love. After all, nothing has meaning unless we put meaning behind it. And if we do not mean what we do, why bother doing it in the first place?

TWO • INGREDIENTS

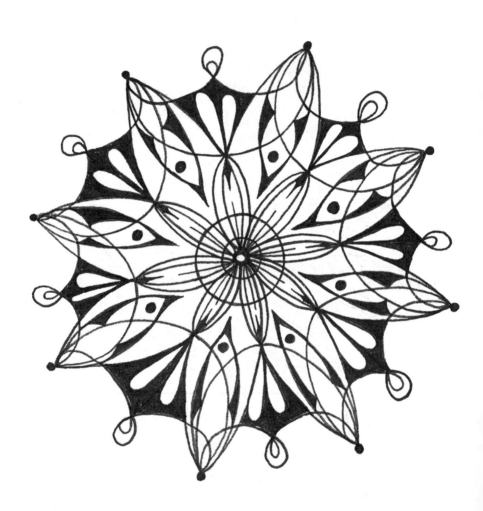

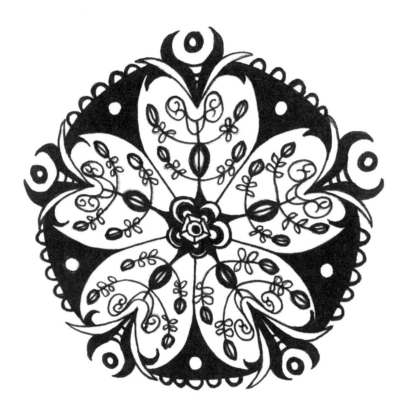

5

Is it an apple or an orange?

Now you are all settled in your body. Your mind is calm. You are present and ready to give your partner a massage. Your partner is lying face down in the prone position. He trusts you and knows that you are going to work with him by being attentive to his verbal and nonverbal cues. Standing on his left side with your feet shoulder-width apart, you rub your hands together and gently place your left hand behind his neck and your right hand over the sheet on top of his sacrum. When he exhales, you increase the contact by increasing the pressure. On the fourth inhalation, slowly raise both hands and move to stand directly in front of him. Your fingertips are making gentle yet firm contact with his scalp – you're not just rearranging his hair and giving him a funky hairdo. When he exhales, you begin moving your fingertips in a circular motion with a combination of small and large circles. All your movements originate from your abdomen, even the tiniest ones, which means when you move your fingers your whole body moves. You are wrapping your middle and ring fingers on each side of his ear with your middle fingers touching his temporal lobes, and continuing to make happy circles there. You are working your way to the base of the head, the occipital, where you find muscles that feel like pebbles. Your happy circles are slowly working their way to minimize the pebbles. You decide you are going to stay there for a little bit longer, keeping your fingertips on top of the muscles, waiting. Your patience turns out to be wise: The pebble-like muscles are getting softer and are now feeling more like tiny grains of sand. With soft fists, you roll your way down to the neck.

Keeping your left hand behind his neck, use your right hand to slowly move the sheet down his back, creating a light brushing on his skin that is gentle and sensual. As you apply lotion with a circular motion, take mental notes on the texture and density of the muscles. Does the muscle feel more like an apple or an orange? An apple's texture is hard and when you

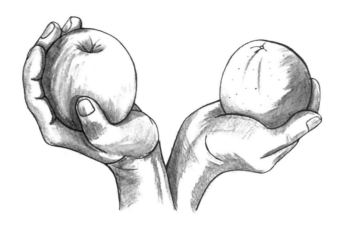

rub your hands over it, it does not yield. An orange, however, can be pressed into and stretched. In the back of your mind, the word "knots" is flashing red. You remember that knots are myofascial trigger points, muscles that are in constant contraction. Ah, yes, the muscles can be as unreasonable as your child and as stubborn as your mom. Funny how parents, babies and muscles act in similar ways sometimes! You start with a gentle negotiation. You follow the muscle fiber direction with the intention of lengthening the "apple." When the apple won't budge, you move to your second strategy, which is to use a cross-fiber technique – if the fiber runs vertically, say, you will work it horizontally. When crossing the fiber, it's good to do so rhythmically. Take advice from the Hendrickson Method: Sync your movements with the heartbeat and move your body like a wave on the ocean. In a rocking motion, use gentle yet persistent pressure, moving your fingers across the fiber at about sixty cycles per minute to the rhythm of the resting heartbeat. The thought is that the constant wave action of the ocean can erode away a mountain. You might not have the ability to turn water into wine but you now have the ability to turn an apple into an orange! After cross-fiber work, go back and follow the fiber direction to soothe the muscle.

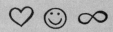

Trick of the Trade

Where to Keep the Massage Lotion
I often take a big plop of lotion and keep it right on my left deltoid, the shoulder's main muscle. Whenever I need extra lotion I have it right on my arm without having to break the massage flow. Some people like to use a massage holster and that works fine too.

Moving your hands back to the base of the neck, glide gently to his mid shoulder blade (scapula) and increase your pressure moving down toward the tailbone (sacroiliac). A lot is happening during this journey. The neck is like a bridge, connecting the head to the shoulders. This bridge is made up of seven cervical vertebrae; with the help of muscles, joints, ligaments and tendons, it is able to perform rotation, flexion and extension. As you cross the bridge, you notice the right side is tighter than the left and you see your partner's right shoulder is pulling toward his ear. You take a detour, resting your palms on top of his shoulders (trapezius) and pushing them toward his feet, one hand at a time, slowly increasing pressure while watching the movement of his body, noticing the left hip has less movement. Go back now between the shoulder blades; they are floating bones with only the collarbone (clavicle) connecting them to the rest of the skeleton. That means the shoulder blades are capable of elevation, depression, protraction, retraction and upward and downward rotation. You are stepping to the right side of his head to give yourself leverage while increasing the pressure between the mid shoulder blades. Your hands are traveling down next to the spine, which is like the central Rocky Mountains. You are moving from the upper back toward the lower back, crossing trapezius to rhomboids and arriving at latissimus dorsi. Upon arrival, you place your hands on top of each other and give the sacrum an extra push toward the feet. Fanning out your fingertips on top of his glutes with your fingers reaching the front of his hip bones (anterior superior iliac joint), grab and pull them slightly toward you. Your hands travel back to each mid scapular, pushing them away from each other, your hands moving back to the top of the shoulders. Once back on the trapezius, push it down toward the feet, and gently move your hands back to the base of the neck. Repeat the journey from the neck to the sacrum a couple of more times, increasing the pressure each time.

On the third visit to the sacrum, you are standing on the right side of his hip, reaching over to slide your right hand on top of his left glutes, pushing the muscle away from the spine,

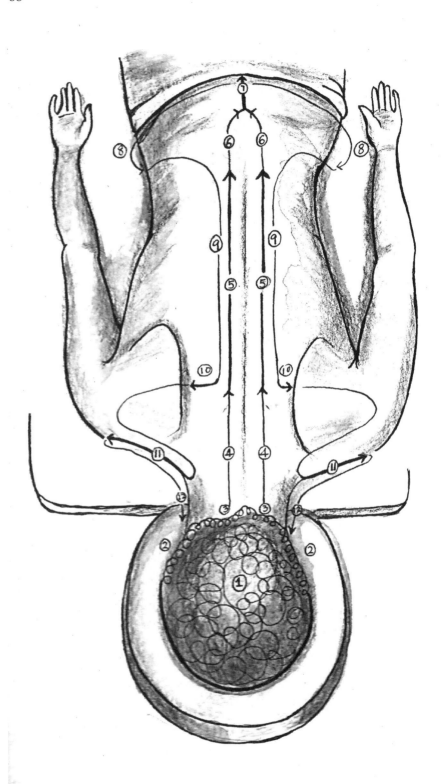

with your left hand following and mimicking the right hand. As you move up on the left side of the rib cage, fan out your fingers so they slide between each rib. The ribs are like ridges and your fingers are traveling down the valleys. Once arriving at the shoulder blade, bring your fingers close together and move over the shoulder blade.

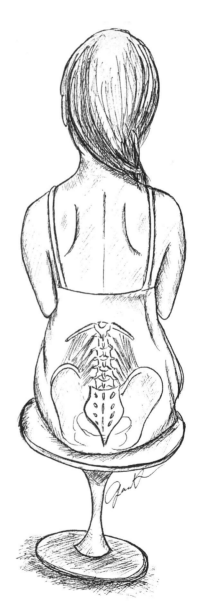

Now embrace the shoulder blade with your right hand on top of the shoulder and your left hand near the armpit, and with your left hand leading the way return to the lower back. Now, instead of pushing the muscles away from the spine, pull them toward it. Once back on the glutes, keep your right hand in place and walk around the table to stand on the left side of your partner.

Give your hands a little break by slowly resting your right elbow on his left gluteus. Check in with your partner on the pressure. With your left hand resting on his sacrum, start to rock his body. This motion generates from you pushing with your right elbow and left hand. The power comes from moving your entire body. You rock, baby! While still in a rocking motion, move your left hand up his back and grab his left shoulder. The right elbow is still pushing but this time the left hand is pulling. This opposing motion creates space and movement on his lower and upper back at the same time. This technique comes from Chinese *Tui Na* massage. *Tui* means pushing and *Na* means grasping. Slow down the rocking motion while bringing your left hand down to the lower back. With your right elbow remaining on the glutes and pushing toward his feet, move your left forearm between the pelvis and the last rib. Now transition the contact from your left forearm to your hand and move it back on the sacrum. Push the sacrum down toward his

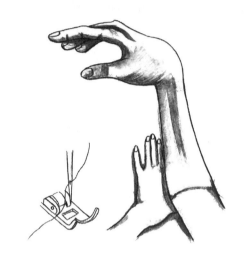

feet and let your right elbow skip and hop over your left hand before you find yourself twisted up, then gracefully lighten up your left hand and leave his sacrum lengthened and happy. Now keep your left fingers together and stretch out your thumb, making an "L" shape with your hand. Slide your right elbow into the L and travel up his back on the erector spinae muscle group right next to the spine. It is a sewing machine where your left hand is the guide and your right elbow is the needle. You are tailoring a bodysuit just for him. As you move up toward his left shoulder blade, ease off on the pressure. Your elbow is following the curve and once on top of the shoulder you slide down next to the neck and move your right arm so your right

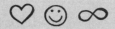

Trick of the Trade

Your Own Massage Tools

Nature provides us with a variety of great massage tools: fingers, knuckles, hands, forearms, elbows, knees, feet and thumbs. Massage therapists tend to start a session with their hands in order to apply lotion and to gain understanding of the body.

We use small tools such as fingers and thumbs for small spaces and delicate areas like the head, face, neck, hands, feet and between the shoulder blades. We also double up the thumbs to create more pressure or place fingers on top of the opposite thumb to increase intensity. Forearms, knuckles and elbows are great tools for broad areas like the back, forearms, glutes, calves and quads.

In some massage practice, like Ashiatsu and some Thai, we use only our feet throughout the entire massage session. We can use our knees for the glutes, since this area can withstand a lot of pressure (and most of us hide our tension there). So play with your tools, and practice to gain sensitivity. Remember, if you cannot feel what you are doing please stop and switch to another tool, and always check in with your partner about applying the right amount of pressure.

hand is now on his shoulder. Together, your hands glide down his left arm and off his body. Now take a breath and shake out your hands.

Breathe in and let both your hands travel up his left fingertips to his arm, reaching his shoulder. Your right hand is grasping his shoulder, your left hand is reaching under it to be in contact with his pectoralis muscle. It is as if there is a magnetic field pulling your left and right hands together while your partner's shoulder is stuck in between. You rocked earlier. Now you are going to roll. You roll his shoulder up and back toward you to open up his chest. Upon finishing the third rolling thunder tour, you slide both your hands to embrace his elbow and bring his arm ninety degrees up toward his head with his forearm draping off the table. Like wringing water from a wet towel, you wring the deltoid, triceps and biceps muscles. Once you reach

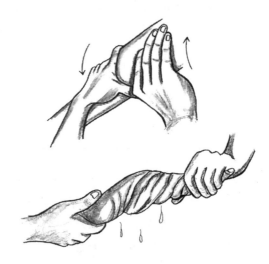

the forearm, you grasp in the middle of the forearm muscles and pull them away from each other to create the stretch, like opening up an orange. Extend your orange-opening skill to the tiny space in the palm. Embrace your hands around his shoulder,

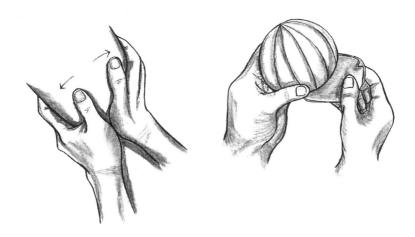

brushing over all the muscles you were just working on, and swing his arm toward his head so now his arm is draping off the table right by his head. Brush your hands from his shoulder to his forearm. Make yourself comfortable by squatting or sitting on the floor. Follow the muscles' direction to lengthen them. Hold his hand in your left hand – by moving the angle of his hand you are able to gain access to different parts of the forearm muscle. Repeat this motion several times. Once his forearm feels like cooked spaghetti noodles, you can move on to his hand. Same idea: Stretch and lengthen each finger and thumb. With your left palm facing up, reach for his elbow and rest his left arm on

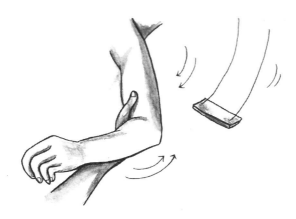

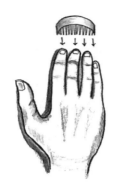

your forearm. This way you are providing complete support and have great control of his arm. Stretch his triceps while his elbow is bent and straighten the arm to stretch the biceps, then go up to his deltoid. Bend his elbow again to place your right fingers next to the spine. Start combing the muscles with your fingers from spine to shoulder blade, all the while swinging his arm from his left to right. The swinging motion opens up the upper back muscles and the combination gives an extra intensity to this very specific stretch.

Over the decade since I started my massage practice, I have only encountered three people who had absolutely no tension in their neck and shoulder. I should have given each one of them a gold medal! The neck and shoulder is like a Bermuda Triangle where you need to navigate with caution or you might mysteriously get lost and experience paranormal activity. The first time I ever trod these waters I was nervous about venturing too far, so I kept my head down, focused three inches in front of my nose, and moved fast like it was a sailboat race. In my head I was thinking, "I am not really sure what I am doing, and I am pretty sure the person on the table doesn't feel good." I was so much in my head that I was making assumptions about what the other person was thinking. You know what assume means right? It is making an ass out of you and me. At that moment I was an ass: I was not present, centered, nor moving with compassion. Instead, I was afraid, embarrassed to ask my partner for feedback and seek assistance from the instructor. So don't be an ass. When I slowed my massage pace I was able to detect the nuances of each muscle, their story and what they wished to unfold, their relationship with each other. The dark, stormy clouds parted

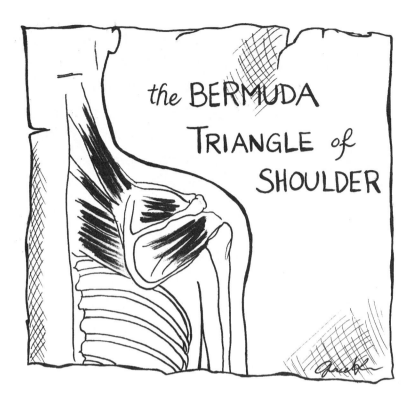

the BERMUDA
TRIANGLE of
SHOULDER

above the Triangle and a silver lining of wisdom shined through.

Gently bring his arm back to his left side, ninety degrees off the table, and do-si-do with his arm by lifting his elbow and gently tossing it between your hands. Slowly relax the elbow on the table. This position opens up the muscles between the spine and shoulder blade nicely. Brush your hands up toward his neck and move to stand in front of him. Your right fingers slide onto the base of his skull (occipital), your left thumb tracing the muscle from the base of his skull to the top of the shoulder. Repeat this move a couple of times and transition to standing on the right side of your partner. With your left and right thumb sitting side by side, lengthen the muscle from spine to shoulder blade at a forty-five-degree angle. You are like an artist sculpt-

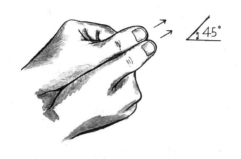

ing a beautiful wing for an angel. Do this move slowly, precisely. This is a healthy place to make a big deal out of something small. Once you are done sculpting, brush from his shoulder to fingers and swing his arm back on the table. This position lands his left palm facing up on the table, a great invitation to give extra care to his thumb. You are going to apply Hendrickson technique here by positioning your body parallel to his thumb. This allows you to work perpendicularly on the thumb. Place your left foot in front of your right with left heel pointing to right toes.

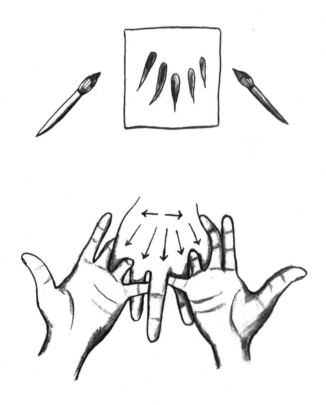

Place your thumbs side by side right off the most meaty part of his thumb (thenar eminence). When you transfer your weight from your right heel to right toes, your body rocks forward and your thumbs move across his thenar eminence. Repeat this until you've worked on this whole area.

Now, with both your palms facing up, lace your right pinky between his middle and ring fingers while your right ring finger slides between his index and thumb. Your left pinky is in between his middle and ring fingers while your left ring finger is in between his ring and pinky. Your fingers are like the wooden frame, stretching and opening up space in his palm, which is like the canvas. Your thumbs are the brushes that are going to paint on the canvas. Right below his wrist, starting in the middle, draw horizontal lines, then draw lines in the tiny space between his bones. Glide your hands from his fingers back to the shoulder. Turn yourself around so you are facing his feet. As your left elbow goes down toward his lower back, your right hand is on his shoulder and glides toward his hand. You find some residual tension in his mid back. Sink into the tension area, going as deep as his body allows you to, and wait patiently. Start shaking your left hand like a rattlesnake to bring ease into

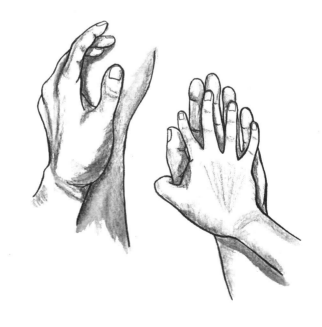

the tense mid back. The shaking helps to distract the mind from the pressure and oftentimes the tensed muscle will go, like two cars driving on different roads at different speeds but arriving at their destination at the same time.

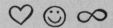

Trick of the Trade

Massage Flow

As my teacher Char Pias describes, imagine your partner's body is a superhighway. You are driving from his right hand up his arm and shoulder, then down his back. You can repeat this loop or keep on driving down his back, glutes and legs, arriving at his right foot. Now if you want to return to his back, you can drive up from his right foot or you can get there from his right hand. To get from right foot to right hand, you will need to make a bridge by touching both body parts at the same time.

This superhighway allows you to travel not only from north to south, but also from east to west, northeast to southwest, and so forth. Going from east to west can be daunting at first, due to the central Rocky Mountains (the spine), but with care you can cross it without a fuss – from any angle. For instance, diagonal body stretching and working feels good to the body. So how do you get to his left shoulder while you are on his right hip? You guessed it, you make a bridge with your hands!

There is no right or wrong way to travel on this superhighway, but it can be awkward if you just stop in the middle of the road and jump to another part of the highway. Once you exit the head, hands or feet, you are welcome to take both your hands off his body. You can take this opportunity to shake out your hands and breathe. There are some schools of thought that your hands should never leave the receiver throughout the massage. However, if your intention is to recharge and refuel before you continue on your journey, a quick break is quite acceptable. Your partner also gets a chance to take in all the changes and shifts in his body.

While you are still standing on his left side, place your right hand on his right glutes and your left hand on his left shoulder blade and stretch them at the same time to create diagonal lengthening. From his left side, you have the perfect opportunity to reach across his body and work on his right side. Work on his glutes with your left hand. Then, moving like a silent ninja, follow with your right hand. Rock his body, tailoring the bodysuit, rolling the shoulder, wringing the wet towel, opening up an orange, making spaghetti noodles, combining the muscle and swinging the arm, do-si-do with the elbow, sculpting the wing, stretching and painting on canvas, rattlesnake, brushing, and gliding down the arm and the back.

Now the tour of the back landscape is about to end, so let's say goodbye to all the places you have just visited. Stand by his right shoulder and glide your hands down his back to his sacrum, pulling your hands back up to his shoulders, down to both arms and hands, moving back up to his shoulders, neck and finally back to his head, where you started.

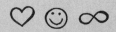

Trick of the Trade

Receiving Massage
Besides relaxing and focusing on your breathing, it is important to speak up when the pressure is too great or weak. Take care, however, to speak kindly and positively to your partner. He is doing his best. Avoid falling into the trap of trying to drive the session and telling him what to do. Remember: "A dream you dream alone is only a dream. A dream you dream together is reality."
~ John Lennon

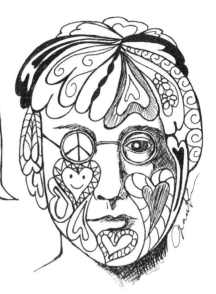

A dream you dream alone is only a dream. A dream you dream together is reality.

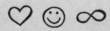

Trick of the Trade

The Art of Doing Nothing

Warm up your hands, cup them over your partner's eyes, and stay there for a minute or two. The contact around the eyes helps the orbicularis, frontal and zygomatic muscles to relax. Cover your partner's ears and let the sound echo and swirl, like the ocean. These two simple moves help relax the body and mind and lift the spirit.

6

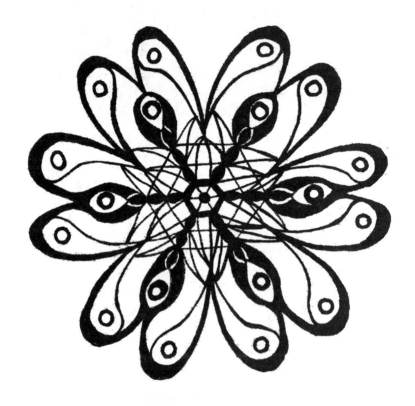

*'The trick to forgetting the big picture is to
look at everything close up.'*
~ Chuck Palahniuk~

Her lower back tension extends to her glutes – no wonder she's been complaining for the last couple weeks about how her back hurts. Now she is on your table in prone position and your hands are finding tight muscles that feel like guitar strings stretched from her twelfth ribs to her pelvis and extending to her glutes. Standing by her right shoulder and facing her feet, you slide your left hand under her right hip bone while your right hand rests on top of her left hip bone. You are preparing to do the twist with her by lifting her right hip and pushing down on her left hip then switching the motion by putting your right hand under her hip and left hand on top. The twist warms up the muscles that you are about to work on. Look

for her right twelfth rib, which is the last rib, and place both your thumbs underneath it, making sure your thumbs aren't just on the surface but sink into the muscle. Your intention is to lengthen this muscle, quadratus lumborum (QL), by pushing the QL down toward the top of the pelvis. After warming up the QL, you go deeper by using rhythmic movement one thumb at a time, moving forward little by little. This movement generates from your hip. Once

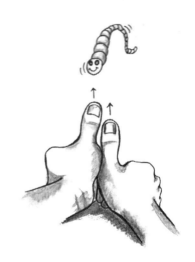

you have reached the top of the pelvis, work your thumbs along the pelvis contour by applying a shiatsu technique. The literal translation for shiatsu is "finger pressure." Place your thumbs side-by-side and press down on the QL when she exhales, then let your thumbs rise when she inhales. Follow her lead, one press at a time, until you can no longer reach. Gently use your hands

84

to brush your way back to where you started the QL work. On the third trip back down to the pelvis, you are going to shiatsu your way there, patiently pressing one inhalation at a time to reach your destination. Go back to the hip twist and move your body to stand by her left shoulder and repeat the lengthening and shiatsu on her left QL. Finish with the hip twist. She takes a really deep breath, sighs, and you see a little twitch in her hands. She is slowly letting go.

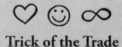

Trick of the Trade

Body Positioning
The position of the receiver's body on the massage table can help to open up areas that need extra lengthening. For example, you can place a pillow underneath the receiver's belly to create extension for his back. And if I were to focus on the right side of his lower back, I would ask him to bring both feet to the left side of the table; in this position, the right side of his lower back is already stretched and opened. One thing I would be extra cautious about is that now his spine is curved to the left, so when I work with the muscle I am following that curve.

Another great body positioning to open up the lower back is to have the receiver kneel down on the massage table, with his forehead touching the table as in Child Position in yoga.

"Why do I need to wait for my partner's exhalation every time when I press down? Shiatsu sounds tediously slow. Wait, is it shiatsu or shih tzu like the dog?"

A classmate once asked this unfiltered question, and I am glad he did, because I was thinking the same thing. As a receiver, I had noticed that when my partner pressed down on my back while I was taking a breath, it felt like I was breathing in against a barrier and my breath was shallow. I also found myself struggling to catch up to and match her pace, instead of her following my lead. It was hard to relax. Giving massage is a lot like making music: the rhythm is our partner's breath, melody is the working hand, harmony is the supporting hand, tempo is the speed you move at when the muscle is relaxed, and subdivision is adding another massage technique while working on a particular muscle. These are basic elements that help in composing beautiful music; once you master these elements, you can build on them and create your own masterpiece.

You move to stand close to her right hip, facing her feet so both your hands are effortlessly in contact with her sacrum. Looking at the sacrum from this direction, it looks like an upright triangle. The sacrum is made up of five fused vertebrae and can withstand quite a lot of pressure. With your palms facing down side by side like a butterfly, push the sacrum toward her feet, stretching and opening up this area. Pressure on a bone doesn't always feel good, but the force on the sacrum helps to open up tiny spaces between each of the fused vertebrae and that feels nice. Hang out there until you feel your partner's tension melting away. Now go deeper at more specific points by using your thumbs. Applying shiatsu technique, sink your thumbs in between the first and second fused vertebrae when she exhales. Let go of the thumb pressure when she inhales and repeat this process a couple more times. Now move on to the space between the second and third fused vertebrae. Stay there for three breathing cycles and move on to the space between the third and fourth fused vertebrae, then the fourth and fifth.

Use loose fists to warm up her right glutes by pressing one fist at a time, a motion that generates from your hip. Here is a great opportunity for you to practice Cirque du Soleil tricks if you are nimble and feeling adventurous. First, gently get on the table with your knees. Second, walk your palms on her glutes. Third, once you are comfortable and confident, switch to one knee on her glutes while keeping your hands on the table to help with balance. Check with her on the pressure – if she would like more pressure, you can use one knee on each glutes. You can

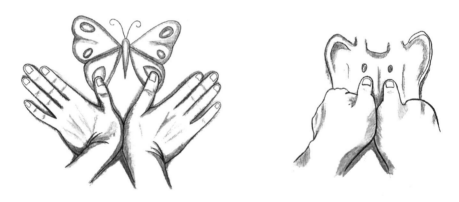

lighten the pressure by transferring weight into your hands and increase the pressure by leaning your weight toward your knees. Slowly and carefully move yourself off the table and with your right elbow, sink into the glutes along the contour of the pelvis, then find the midpoint of her glutes and press down there. You are being careful and yet firm here because your elbow is now on her piriformis, which is right above her sciatic nerve. Once you feel the muscle starting to melt, move your right elbow straight down the mid gluteus and place it at the point where glutes meet leg. Now you are on the hamstring attachment site. With your left hand, reach over to grab her right heel and stretch. Gracefully undrape her right leg up to her glutes and gently tug the sheet under. Take a look at how her feet are resting on the table. Are her heels turning inward, outward or lining up straight with her hip? Warm up lotion in your hands and glide up her leg, making only very gentle contact when reaching behind her knee. Slowly increase the pressure as you go up the glutes on the way back down her foot by simply stepping back, moving your body, and dragging your hands with you. Like a master calligrapher holding a giant brush, you want every movement to come from your center – your arms and legs move with your body. On your second trip up to visit the glutes, use your right hand and left forearm. Your right hand leads the way with gentle pressure and your forearm follows with firm pressure. At her gluteus, your left forearm glides and moves to let the left elbow contact the gluteus instead. Move the elbow toward the middle of the gluteus. You are back on her piriformis again. Stay there and move the right hand onto her lower back and wait for a softening. Follow the curve toward the outside of the hip and eventually drop down to the side of the thigh. Here is her iliotibial band (ITB), which is a thin layer of fascia, so go gently. The elbow is leading the way back down toward the knee and the right hand is brushing down the ITB. Upon reaching the middle of the hamstring, move the elbow across it and glide down toward the knee and embrace the knee with both your hands. Your thumbs are side by side at the midline of her calf. Step back and bring both your arms and her calf with you when you reach her ankle. Create a gentle traction by supporting the front of her ankle with your left hand and her heel with your right hand. Turn your right hand into a soft fist and use the knuckles to work your way down the foot, then go up the leg and glutes one more time before getting ready to stretch her leg.

Grab her right foot with your hands, bend her knee ninety degrees, then brace her ankle with your thumbs and index fingers. With your feet rooted in the ground, gently lift her leg off the table and rock it; notice how the movement travels up to her mid back. This opens up the hip nicely. Very gradually bring the rocking to a stop. With the knee still bent, relax it back on the table. While her foot is still in your hands, begin moving her toes to open up space between them. With your fingers at the midline on the ball of her foot, grasp and pull the muscles outward, working your way down the whole foot, like peeling an orange. Rest your left hand on her right heel with your forearm resting on her foot and push your forearm down to stretch her calf; her Achilles tendon is also getting a good stretching. Your right thumb and index finger make downward circles from her heel to the Achilles. Grasping her big toe and supporting the arch of her foot and shaking, you see her calf muscles are moving freely. Slowing down the shaking, place your right hand on her lower back and stretch the foot toward her gluteus. This gives her quadriceps a good stretching. You noticed that she is very flexible so you keep her foot down toward the gluteus with your right hand while your left hand moves underneath her knee and lifts it up. She feels the stretch all the way up to her hip and lower belly. You remember to take your time here, listening to her body and waiting for the release. At the same time, you are checking in with your own body. "Am I standing comfortably? Is my body aligned? Are my face and shoulders relaxed?"

Moving your left hand to support her foot, keep the knee bent ninety degrees and make a soft fist on her gluteus with your right hand. Bring her foot toward you and push down on her

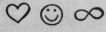

Trick of the Trade

Three Times the Charm

Massaging an area three times is not the Golden Rule, but it is a great way to introduce massage pressure and give a receiver's body time to warm up, let go, and relax. It is like going out with someone for the first time – you shake hands, exchange a polite hug, maybe a kiss on the cheek. On the second date, you want to know more about each other, so you ask questions to find out about their past and present and their plans for the future. On the third date, you let go of your defenses, melt into each other's arms, and passionate kisses follow.

gluteus at the same time. This stretches her piriformis and provides a deep opening for her hip. Now here comes the fun part – the Frog Leg Stretch. You are standing at her feet, facing her. With your right hand under her knee and your left hand on her foot, lift her right leg by resting her foot on your shoulder. Legs can be heavy, so don't be shy about putting your whole body into the lifting. Now gently bring her knee out to the right and

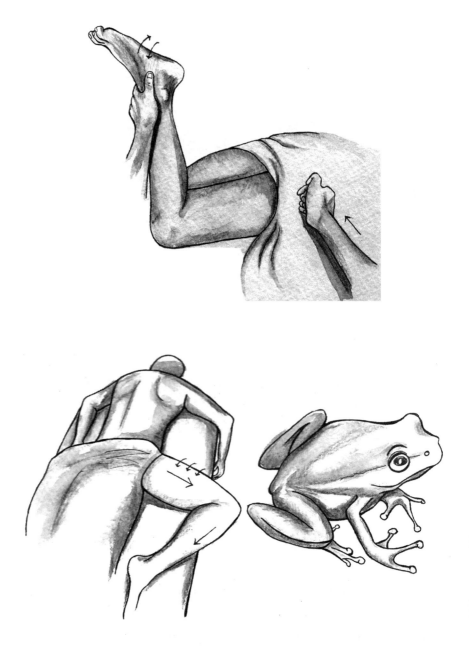

rest the leg on the table. The frog position gives you easy access
to her ITB, part of her quads and the muscle outside the shin
(tibialis anterior), and at the same time stretches her inner thigh,
warming up the muscles from her foot to ITB and the side of

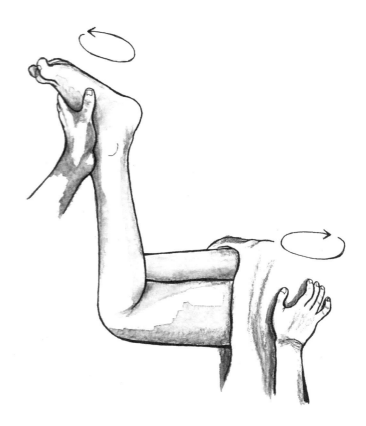

her hip. Remember, the ITB is sensitive, so go easy on it, lacing your fingers together and using your palms as you move from her knee to her hip. Check in with her on the pressure and adjust accordingly. Use your fingers like teeth, grasping and combing the quads from the inner thigh toward the ITB, skipping over the knee and landing your finger teeth on the tibialis anterior. The pretend teeth are glued together and moving up and down the muscle. Once at the foot, get a firm hold of it with your left hand while your right hand supports the knee, and swing the knee back on the table. With the knee still bent, move your right palm onto her gluteus, your fingers in contact with her sacrum, and rotate her foot counterclockwise. You're pressing down on her gluteus and moving your right hand clockwise at the same time.

Moving large limbs, especially large legs, is intimidating for someone who is petite and slim like me. My partner in one class was a big guy – his leg was the size of my body! He seemed to notice my hesitation, so he moved his own leg to the side for the frog leg stretch. "Thank God!" I thought. "But I really wanted to learn how to do it without his help." I wished I was Vishnu with great strength and multiple arms. Needless to say, my wish was not granted. Instead we adjusted the table to a lower height, allowing me to use my core muscles to do the lifting. Using only my shoulders and arms was exhausting and unsafe. My teacher asked me to pay attention to the alignment of my body and reminded me to ground my feet before I lifted, techniques that made a significant difference. I was able to ease into the move without hurting myself. That said, if his leg was any heavier, I would have asked him to please move to the side in order to avoid injury.

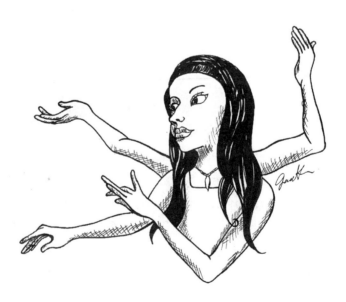

Trick of the Trade

Massage Without a Massage Table

Shiatsu and Thai massage are both practiced on the floor. Your rhythm of massage matches your partner's breath: Lean your weight into her when she exhales and bring your weight back toward your glutes when she inhales. Remember what Dr. Seuss says? "Life's a Great Balancing Act. Just never forget to be dexterous and deft. And never mix up your right foot with your left."

Thai massage teacher Rachel Johnson says she often has her husband sit on the floor while she sits on the couch behind him, a position that makes it easy for her to work on his neck and shoulders. She can lean in on a shoulder with her forearm using a rolling pin motion, or use her elbow for more pressure without any effort. Ah, again it is the art of doing nothing.

Another Thai technique has the giver in the lotus position, back against a wall, pillow resting on his lap, and the receiver's head on the pillow. This semi-reclining position is comforting for the receiver and provides the giver easy access to the face, neck and shoulders. Massage can also be done on a chair. When I visited my family in Taiwan a couple of months ago, I had my dad sit facing the back of a chair; although his arms were unsupported, this worked pretty well as a makeshift massage "table."

All the excitement of the flying leg is about to come to an end. You are preparing for landing by supporting the foot with your left hand and your right hand on her hamstrings. Slowly drop her foot down on the table and press down on the hamstring at the same time. Repeat until you cover the whole hamstring and gracefully trace over the foot, then let go.

Undrape the whole right side of her body so you are able to glide from her foot to her shoulder and down her arm without obstruction. On the second round your right hand is leading and your left forearm is following. Glide back from her arm to shoulder, turn to face her foot, your right forearm gliding down her back while your left hand moves down her arm at the same time. Forearm and hand meet together at the gluteus and move down the leg together. The third time is just the same, except when the forearm and hand meet at the gluteus, the right hand goes back up to the shoulder and the left hand goes down the leg. Your right hand arrives at her hand and your left hand reaches her foot at the same time. Drape the right side of her body. Using loose fists, move from her right foot to left foot by shifting your weight from the right to the left. Find a nice rhythm that you can relax into. Use this time to stretch your body and check in with how you are feeling. Now you are going to make the transition to work on the left side of her body.

With your right hand on her left foot, your left hand makes a bridge reaching over to her left glutes. Use two loose fists, rhythmically warm up the gluteus muscles, then sink your left elbow into them by following the contour of the hip. Move into the middle of the gluteus, then straight down to where the gluteus and leg meet – the attachment of the hamstring – while your right hand reaches over to her left foot and stretches it. Slowly undrape her left leg up to her gluteus and get ready to do

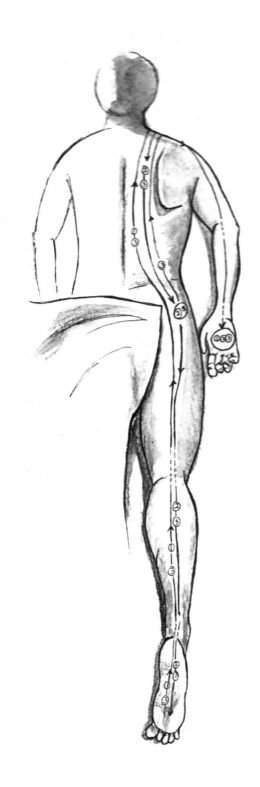

the flying leg routine. Start with a giant calligraphy brush warming up the leg muscle, then follow by applying more pressure with your forearm. On the way down the leg you work gently on her ITB with the side of your elbow. Repeat it one more time to relax the leg.

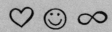

Trick of the Trade

Surrender
Opposite motion and different massage strokes make it hard for the receiver to anticipate, and oftentimes the mind just checks out, letting go of control.

Bend her knee to ninety degrees, embrace the ankle, lift, and shake to open the hip. You then stretch her toes, foot and Achilles tendon, shaking the calf muscle. Push her foot toward her gluteus and lift her knee to increase the stretch. Push into the glutes while bringing her leg out toward the left side to stretch the piriformis. Frog Leg Stretch by lifting the leg up and swinging the knee out toward the left to gain access to her outside leg muscles. Work on her ITB, comb her quads, and slide up and down the tibialis anterior with finger teeth. Bring the knee back on the table, right hand supporting the foot, left hand on the gluteus, and draw two opposite circles with your hands. Push down on the hamstring, resting the foot on the table until you cover the whole hamstring, slide down the calf, and eventually let go of contact once reaching her foot. Undrape her entire left side, first borrowing the calligrapher's brush to glide from foot up to shoulder, down the arm and one more time with forearm. Go down the back with left forearm, right hand down the arm, meeting at the glutes and going down the leg together. Repeat the move one more time and once at the glutes, turn into a gentle giant with your left and right hand going opposite directions. Your left hand ends in her hand and your right hand on her foot.

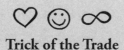

Trick of the Trade

Work Locally and Think Globally

It is easy to focus on a single area of the body and become so absorbed you find yourself almost nose to nose with the muscle you are working on. Be careful – it's important to pay attention to the receiver's whole body. Take mental notes on any twitch, shake, tensing of a muscle, or releasing of tension. Remember, too, to check in with your own body: If you are tensing up during a massage session, the same tension can be transferred to the receiver energetically.

Cover her up now, brushing your hands from her feet up toward the sacrum, and keep your right hand on the sacrum while your left hand continues up the spine to the back of her neck. As your right hand makes circles on her sacrum, rub her neck with your left hand. Then your right hand joins your left hand, together rubbing the neck. Step to stand behind her head and with both hands, work from neck to scalp and make happy circles with your fingers before slowly coming to a stop. Move hands away physically and then energetically.

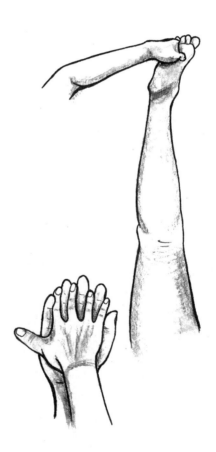

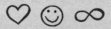

Trick of the Trade

Bigger than Life Sensation

During a massage session with Eric, my hands were moving the opposite direction starting from his waistline and ending one hand in his hand and the other hand on his foot. He later told me it felt as if I were a giant, covering his whole body in one single massage stroke. He wasn't the only person who felt like I transformed into a Hulk-like creature – though not the sort about to smash things. It feels good to have a gentle giant massaging your back and legs once in a while.

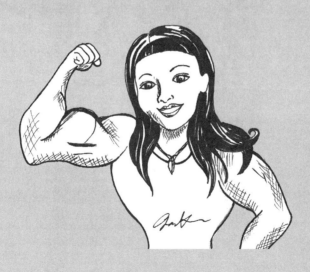

7

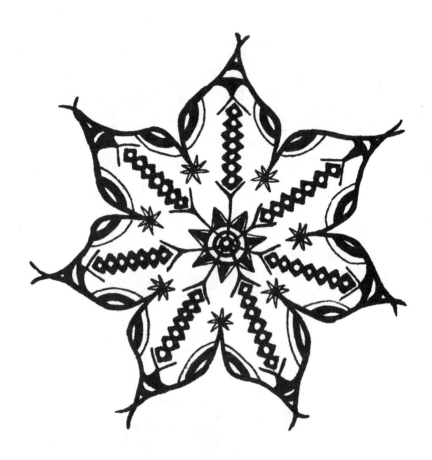

'But the eyes are blind. One must look with the heart.'
Antoine de Saint-Exupéry, The Little Prince

Your partner is lying on his back facing the sky. He is in supine position. Continue massaging his head and take a moment to look at his face. Is he frowning or smiling? Is his head aligned with his body or turned to one side? Check in with your body. Are you aligned? And what about your breathing, is it pleasant? If you did not have time to brush your teeth after eating garlic, onion, curry, chili five-spice stew with melted goat cheese, it might be a good idea to pop in a breath mint. Gently lay your hands on top of his head with your thumbs lying side by side on his forehead, right above his eyebrows, and your fingers cradling the side of his head without covering his ears. Increase your pressure slightly until you feel a slight resistance. The feeling here is as if your thumbs are melting into his head and your intention is to move ever so slightly when there is a release. Move like a snail, see if you can spend five minutes moving your thumbs toward his temporal lobes. This technique is a little taste of myofascial release, and oftentimes the slow pace takes the mind into the subconscious realm. Place your laced fingers on his mid forehead and slowly pull your fingers apart to draw three lines toward his temporal lobes. Once there, make circles with your index, middle, and ring fingers. Keep the contact with temporal lobes, bring your thumbs back to the middle of the forehead, and trace those three lines again, one at a time, starting with the one close to the hairline. Gently rest your thumbs on the tip of his nose and glide over it, then pause the thumbs right above the eyebrows. Starting on the side of each nostril, move your index fingers upward, following the contour of the nose to the brow, fingers joining the thumbs, two soft lips gently kissing the brows until you reach the temporal lobes, or "temples."

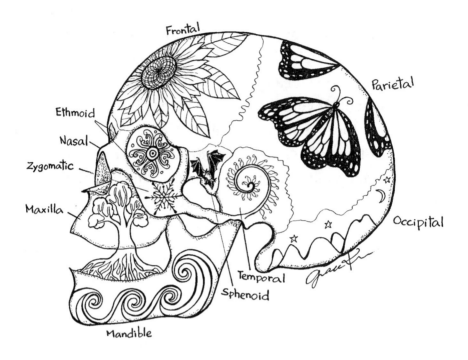

Now get ready to draw the "Infinity Glasses."

With your right index and middle fingers, trace under the right eye orbit, moving up across the nose ridge and tracing above the left eyebrow ridge, then traveling down to the left temple continue under the left eye orbit across the nose ridge, curving above the right eyebrow ridge and arriving back where you started, at the temple. Massage the right temple in a circular motion, then bring the left fingers into the rhythm on the opposite temple, preparing to draw the glasses starting from the left side: under the left eye orbit, across the nose, above the right eyebrow ridge, under the right eyebrow ridge, across the nose, above the left eyebrow and back at the left temple. Make happy circles there and let the right temple join the party.

In succession, like playing the piano, the index fingers followed by middle, ring and pinky go to the side of the nostril, below the cheekbones. Now, to find his temporomandibular joints (TMJs), ask your partner to open and slowly close his mouth. Glide your fingers there and make happy circles. The right TMJ feels tighter under your fingers, so ask him to slowly open his jaw as you move your fingers from the joint toward his chin and underneath the cheekbones. You are on his chewing muscle, the masseter. Pound for pound, this is the strongest muscle in the human body and can take a good amount of pressure. Work firmly from underneath the cheekbone toward the jaw to smooth

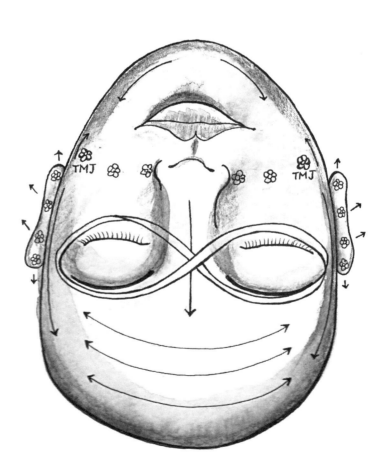

and stretch the muscle in order to relax his TMJ. Thumbs go right in the middle of the jaw line and fingers support the chin, tracing the curve up toward the TMJ.

Now lace your fingers under his chin and trace the contour of his face upward. Your fingers arrive at the TMJs while thumbs move up the nose bridge toward the third eye and fingers continue on toward the temples. Together, your fingers and thumbs are heading toward his hairline, massaging the scalp with a combination of small and large circles. Explore the area behind the ears. With thumbs at the midline of the chin, lace your fingers under it and repeat the manual "facelift" a couple of more times.

Land your thumbs on his third eye and slide right to where the eyebrows begin, index fingers on both sides of the

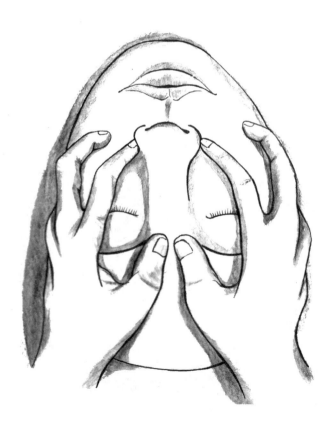

nose, middle fingers underneath the middle of the cheek bone, ring fingers bent to place on the temples, pinkies reaching for the TMJs. This finger placement, looking like a variation on the Vulcan Mind Meld, was introduced by Kenneth Kole (Kole the craniosacral acupressure teacher, not Cole the fashion designer). This position facilitates the balance of all twelve meridians at the same time – "Beauty Mask" is an appropriate description. Holding acupressure points requires patience, which means you need to be sitting comfortably in your body, present and with a quiet mind, listening for the pulse in all the points and waiting for synchronicity. You may find it can be harder to be still than to move around, so take a deep breath and remind yourself that this is a great opportunity to meditate and be content in the moment.

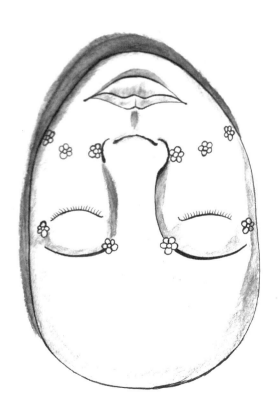

Gently remove your fingers from his face when he inhales. Move to his ears and lightly rub and pull on them – you will now apply acupressure technique in a particular sequence taught in Janet Oliver's Five Elements acupressure class for releasing shoulder and neck tension. Remain seated behind your partner and, starting with your palms facing up, slide your middle fingers underneath his shoulder bilaterally. Moving above the armpit crease, you are at SI (Small Intestine) 9, *Upright Shoulder*. Move your middle fingers about four fingers above the last point

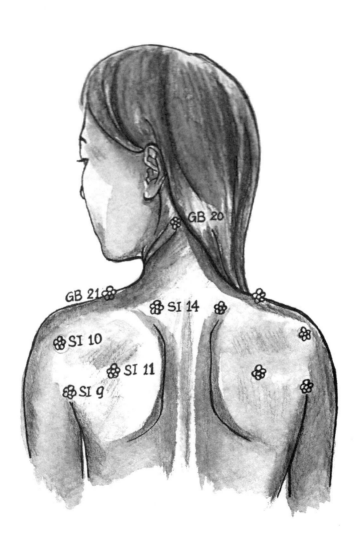

and sink in. You are on SI 10, *Upper Arm Shu*. Find the middle of his shoulder blade and rest there. This is SI 11, *Celestial Gathering*. Eyes closed, you detect delicate changes in his body. Your hands become more sensitive to muscle tissue texture, in tune with his pulse. You feel the rise and fall of his weight above your hands. You breathe with him and detect the same area in your body. You are quietly and simply noticing his body and yours, without judgment.

Move on to SI 14, *Outer Shoulder Shu*, which is on the back, above the inner edge of the shoulder blade on the line lateral to the lower border of the spinous process of the first thoracic vertebrae. Wait until the pulse syncs and move your thumbs along on top of the trapezius to find the middle point. You are on GB (Gallbladder) 21, *Shoulder Well*. Next: *New Recognition*, about midway down the back of the neck, two fingers' width from the neck central line on the outer edge of the muscle band. The last point is GB 20, *Wind Pool*, at the base of the skull in the hollows.

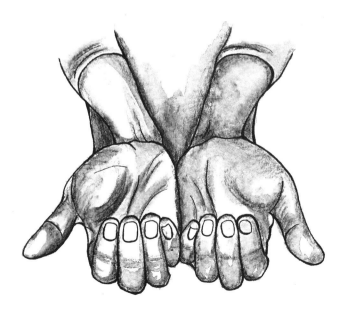

When working with acupressure point, intention is vital, because energy follows intention. Pressing hard on the points is not the point.

Slide your hands to the base of the skull and lift up his head so your fingertips are supporting the weight. Your fingertips are in contact with deep neck muscles, but your partner controls how deep you go by how much he lets go. Instead of push and pull, you are patiently waiting and listening. This technique, called CV4 from Upledger CranioSacral Therapy, takes patience, lots of patience, for your partner to completely let go the control of his neck muscles. You see him resisting at first, with eyes wide, wondering what you are doing, so you speak calmly and remind him that he is in charge and there is no rush. You encourage him to imagine the front of his neck getting longer and more relaxed with every exhalation. His head moves to the right, then slowly toward the center, and you feel the weight increase and your fingertips sinking deeper. More waiting and listening until finally his whole head rests in your palms. CV4 is intense work for the receiver, requiring trust – the "Hurry up and relax!" model does not fit in here.

I had a fight recently with a dear friend of mine. It was so awful that I wanted to end the work day early and head straight home to hide in my bed. How could I focus on making other people feel good when I was feeling lousy? Bad feelings were overtaking me, I was drowning in wave after wave of self-doubt. The massage room was occupied with my sadness. Then I remembered to take my own advice, starting by focusing on the breath and filling my mind with happy thoughts. Like in Harry Potter when he needed to defeat the Dementors: He had to think of the happiest moment in his life to conjure the Patronus Charm. Instead of saying "expecto patronum!" I tuned in to the cranial rhythm of my client by quieting my mind and focusing my attention on him. His rhythm brought me peace. After the session ended I thought to myself, "Wow, this thing really works!" The peaceful space allowed me to reflect on the argument and gave me the emotional capacity I needed to view the mess from new perspectives. Later, my friend and I were able to make up and discuss how idiotically irrational we were.

Bring your hands underneath the neck with index fingers contacting the cervical vertebrae and the rest of the hands there to support the weight of the neck. Each index finger takes turns leading the stretch. Start with the right index gently pulling on the base of the neck (C7) toward his head, landing in the gap between C7 and C6. You see his head tilt slightly to the left. Your left index moves forward, moving the right index out of the way and taking over its spot. Now his head is tilting slightly to the right. Go one cervical vertebra at a time, moving all the way up to the base of the skull. It is like your index fingers are playing hide-and-seek. You are essentially rolling your index fingers from where the neck and body meet, toward the head. This lands

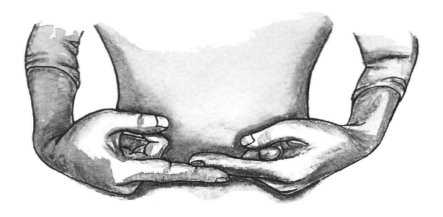

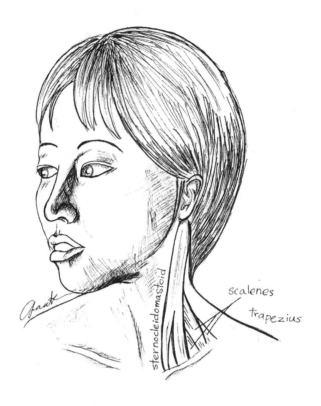

sternocleidomastoid

scalenes

trapezius

you in the perfect position for neck stretching. Lift his head off the table with both your hands and bring his head toward his left shoulder, keeping his nose pointing to the sky until you

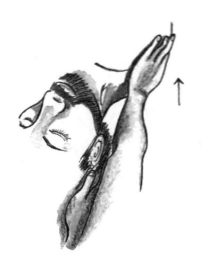

reach a point of resistance. Then rest his head back on the table and with your right hand supporting the head like an anchor, push down on his right shoulder with your left palm. You are crossing your arms to stretch his trapezius. While your left palm traces a path from his shoulder to his neck, make a soft fist with your right hand, palm facing down – as if you were holding an egg – and trace the muscle from the base of the neck back to the shoulder. Repeat the move a couple of more times, each time increasing the pressure slightly. Keep his head resting on the table and slowly turn his head to the left, so his nose is now facing left. Make sure that his ear is not folded. Make happy circles from the base of his head (occiput), up behind his ears, circling on his temple and back down to the occiput. His levator scapula, which helps him to raise his shoulder, is in plain view. The levator scapula runs from the neck to the inside top corner of the shoulder blade. With your soft, egg-holding fist, trace the muscle and find the spot on top of the shoulder blade that is tighter than the rest. Slowly sink your thumb in there. Keep your thumb on that spot nice and steady while your left hand lifts the head and moves his chin toward his left nipple. This increases the intensity of the stretch, so wait patiently until you feel the softening under your thumb, then rest his head back on the

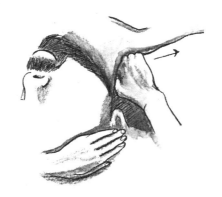

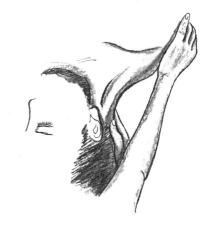

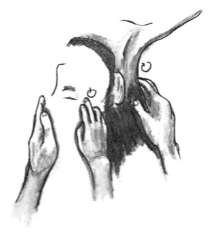

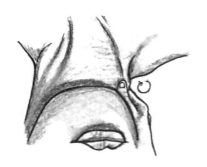

table in neutral position by aligning his head with the rest of his body. Turn his head so his nose is now pointing to the right. Ask him to lift up his head slightly so you can see his sternocleido-mastoid (SCM) muscle, popping out to say hello. With his head still supported in your left hand, turn to the right and grab his SCM with your thumb and index finger; with this motion, like twisting to close a bottle cap, you are working the whole SCM. When the front of the neck muscles tighten, they tend to rotate medially toward the throat. Twisting and closing the cap – a shearing motion – goes in opposition to this, helping to stretch the tight muscle.

Keep his head turned to the right. Find his scalenes muscle by sliding your thumb right behind the SCM. Feel the scalenes with your fingers and trace the muscles from the base of the head (occiput) toward the collarbone (clavicle). You want to slowly warm the region. Think of it like spreading a stick of cold butter on the neck – it takes time, but with repetition, the cold chunks eventually soften and melt. Now that the neck is

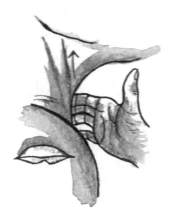

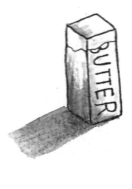

nicely buttered, to make the perfect PB&J sandwich (What, you don't put butter on your PB&J?) align his head with the rest of his body and spread the peanut butter on the scalenes until it is nicely covered. Turn his head by pointing his nose to the left and cover the scalenes with jelly. Bring his delicious neck back to a

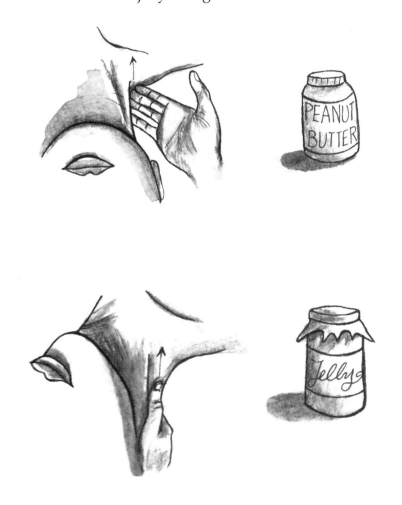

neutral position, pause for a couple seconds, then lift his head and move it to the right. It's time to give the left side of his neck the same love and attention, starting by anchoring his head with your left hand and stretching his shoulder with your right. Use the soft-egg fist to work on the trapezius and turn his nose to face right, making happy circles from occiput to tempo, sliding back to occiput, egg fist on levator scapula. Find the tension spot, sink your left thumb in, and lift his head up by pointing his chin toward his right nipple. When you sense the softening, bring his head back to a neutral position, then slowly turn it to the left. Locate his SCM and apply the twist-and-open-the-cap motion to the whole muscle, moving behind the SCM to locate the scalenes. Use the spreading-butter technique to cover the muscles, then rotate his head to neutral position and this time put on some peanut butter. Once satisfied, turn his head to the right and cover the scalenes with jelly. Relax the head back to neutral. Now, with two egg-holding fists you will turn the right wrist clockwise and the left one counter-clockwise at the same time, imagining you

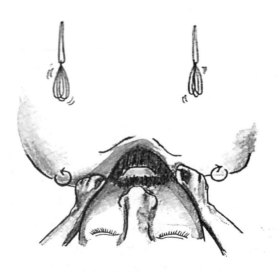

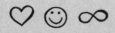

Trick of the Trade

Working with the Neck
The neck is full of delicate nerves and blood vessels, such as the vagus nerves and jugular vein, so it is important to practice on your own neck and feel pressure sensations before working on your partner. As a receiver, communicate with your partner in case there is any tingling sensation or discomfort. If tingling occurs, adjust your finger placement slightly to slide away from the nerve. Don't be afraid to work on the neck – the journey might seem intimidating, but you will surely find hidden treasures.

are making scrambled eggs. You are beating the eggs starting from the base of the neck toward the shoulder and back to the neck, and you are repeating the wrist rotation until everything is nice and fluffy.

Standing with one leg in front of the other, bend your knees so you are almost at the same height as the massage table. Push on your partner's shoulders one at a time by shifting your weight from one foot to the other. Check in with your own body to see if your back is tensing up – you can take this opportunity to stretch a bit. Your fingers should be spread out and angled so they are pushing on his pectoralis muscles toward his sternum on exhalation. Keep your hands on the sternum and pause for a couple of breathing cycles. On inhalation, draw your hands up toward the clavicles and push down in the space between the clavicle and first rib on exhalation. Make three dots down each side of the pectoralis muscles, until you arrive just above the nipples. Remember the connecting the dots game? It's just like that! Again, spread your fingers and push down on the pectoralis muscles when he exhales, then with your fingertips brush

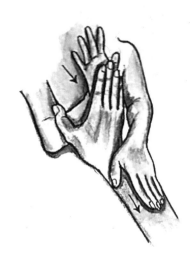

from the sternum toward his right shoulder, down the arm, and out his fingertips. Make contact with his fingers and move up toward his wrist. Once there, gently lift with your thumbs and index fingers, pulling his hand toward his feet to create traction. Keeping his hand on the table with palm facing down, each time you lift his fingers to reveal his palm with your right hand, your left hand will press down on his forearm and push up toward his elbow to create a pumping motion. Lift and glide until his whole forearm gets a good workout. Holding his hand in the handshake position, squeeze the forearm with your left thumb, index and middle fingers while turning his wrist to increase the sensation. Lace your fingers with his palm facing yours and bring his elbow to ninety

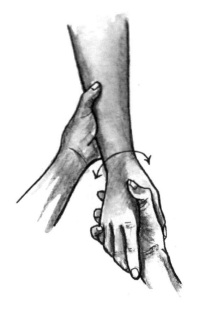

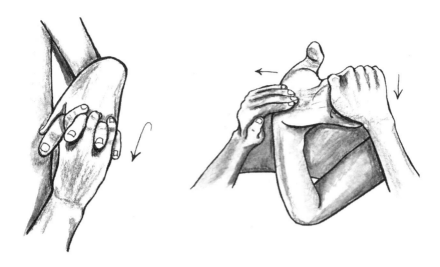

degrees. Brace his wrist with your left thumb and index finger and rotate the wrist. Dig your fingertips between his knuckles to stretch his fingers. Rest his elbow on the table while your left hand stretches his fingers to keep the palm open, facing the sky, and your right fingertips comb the palm. Keep his palm open and tilt his elbow up to face the sky with help from your right hand so his palm is touching the table right by his head. This move opens up all the muscles in his palm and triceps, and also

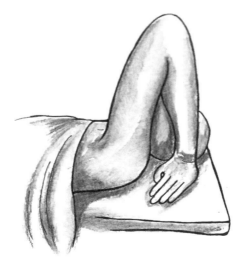

opens up the right side of the ribs. Anchoring his elbow with your left hand, with your right hand glide from his elbow toward the armpit to work on the triceps. Support his whole arm in your left arm and reach under his right lower back with your right hand. Let his weight create the pressure that allows your fingers to sink into his back muscles. Scoop your fingers up toward his upper back and slide over his arm with your right palm in his and your left thumb and index finger bracing his wrist, then step back and stretch his arm over his head. Repeat the tricep, back and overhead stretch a couple more times.

Gently bring his hand down toward his shoulder and bend his elbow, and while holding his hand in arm-wrestle position drop the elbow on the table so the forearm and elbow form a ninety degree angle. With his hand still in yours, turn to face his feet. Your left fingertips are getting ready to comb his pectoralis by finding the groove that is right next to the shoulder and right below the clavicle. Your left fingers are combing from groove to sternum while your right hand is stretching his hand toward his

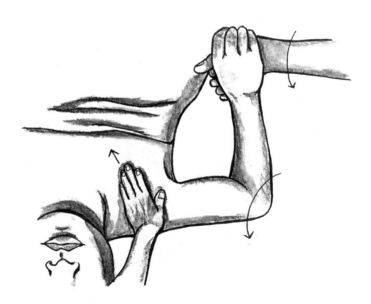

head. There is a slight tension in his pectoralis, so you take the time to sink into the muscle and wait until it starts to soften under your fingertips. Repeat the stretching and combing once or twice more to communicate to the muscle that it is OK to let go.

With his hand still in yours, and the elbow and forearm still at ninetydegrees, move to stand parallel to his shoulder. As your left hand grabs his deltoid, bring his hand down toward his feet. Meanwhile with your left hand pretend to peel the deltoid off his shoulder by grasping and pulling it toward his head. Lift his arm with a gentle shaking motion, then bring it back down to the table, brace his wrist, and stretch his arm toward his feet. Brush up his arm and move to stand behind his head, pushing down on his shoulders one at a time with the last contact on his left shoulder. Brush down his left arm, supporting his wrist and

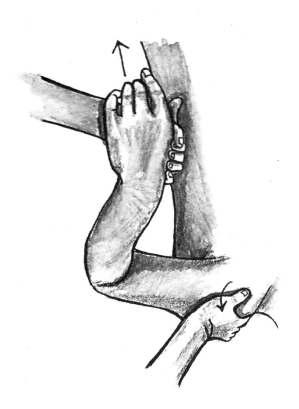

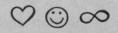

Trick of the Trade

Applying Hot and Cold Therapy

While I was working at Spa Equinox in San Mateo I picked up this neat trick from Maggie Keber, the aesthetician: Roll up four face towels and one hand towel and soak them in hot water with a drop of lavender or peppermint essential oil.

After massaging the back, wipe down one side of the body with a hot face towel and leave the towel on the hand then repeat on the other side. Next, with another face towel, wipe down one side of the lower back down to the foot, leaving the towel on the foot. Repeat on the other side. The heat is comforting and grounding in the hands and feet (this is an operating concept in hot stone massage, as well).

Remove the towels before the client turns over to a supine position. After a great face, neck and shoulder massage, place the hot hand towel under the neck. Of course, check in with your partner on the temperature. Place cold cotton balls over closed eyelids, which will feel extremely refreshing and reduce any puffiness.

gently pulling on it to create traction, then open up his palm by lifting his fingers while pushing and gliding on his forearm from wrist to elbow. Pinch the forearm from elbow to wrist while rotating his hand.

Now bend his elbow to ninety degrees. While supporting the wrist and rotating his hand, stretch his fingers to open up his palm, then comb the palm with your fingertips. Keep the palm open and reach up to the ear and touch the table with it. Working from elbow toward armpit, slide on the side of his left ribs to reach under his waistline, and then once you have contact with his lower back scoop your hand up toward his arm. Hold his hand in your hands and stretch it overhead. Repeat the tricep work, scooping the back and stretching overhead a couple of more times. With his elbow resting on the table, swing the arm back toward the ear, then stretch his hand toward his head while combing his pectoralis at the same time. Bring his arm parallel to his shoulder with his elbow still on the table, and stretch his arm down toward the feet while peeling his deltoid toward his head. Finally, bring the elbow down and stretch the arm toward the feet.

Gently glide your hands up his left arm while facing him, with your left hand on his left shoulder and your right hand on his right shoulder. Alternate pushing down on the shoulders, glide over his pectoralis, then rest your hands on his sternum. Sync your breathing pattern with his and on inhalation, slide your fingers up to his neck, chin, cheek and forehead before landing gracefully on his head. His smile lets you know that your happy circles on the scalp are creating a welcome sensation.

8

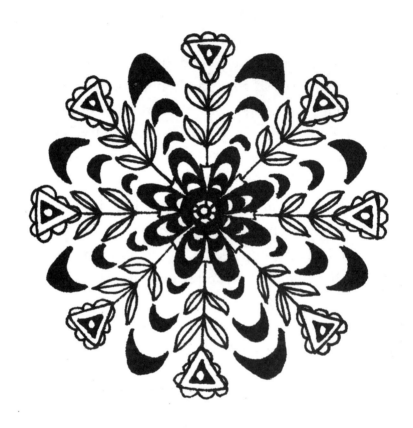

'We're never so vulnerable as when we trust someone
- but paradoxically, if we cannot trust,
neither can we find love or joy.'
~Walter Anderson~

Cover your partner's chest area with a hand towel, slide the sheet down so it is just above her pubis, and tug the sheet under her hip. Stand on her right side facing her belly button and warm up your hands by rubbing them together. Gently make contact with her by sliding your right hand from her left waistline to the intimate, vulnerable, sacred space that is between the belly button and pubis. *Dan Tien,* the Chinese call it, *Hara* in Japanese. Both cultures believe this is where we store our life energy. Your left hand should be moving from her right waistline to land right above the belly button. Your hands are radiating warmth and love. You can feel her breath under your hands. When she inhales, your left hand rises and your right hand follows. When she exhales, your left hand and then right hand sink into her. On the next breathing cycle you close your eyes to feel the expansion of her abdomen. In your mind's eye you see an ocean wave. Her inhalation and exhalation are like the wind. You dive in deeper to explore her ocean, this mysterious body of water. "What lies within?" you ask yourself silently. "What emotion does she hold in here?" Her inhalation is a cue to start drawing clockwise circles with your hands from small to

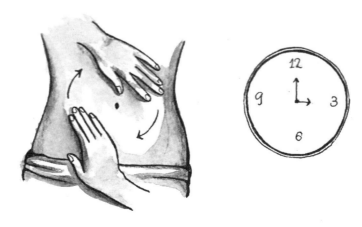

large, using her belly button as the focal point. Move your right hand toward her stomach and your left hand to her abdomen, right hand jumping over the left hand before they collide. When you reach the outer border of her ocean, place your left hand on top of your right, going deeper by pressing your fingers down when she exhales. Like an elegant diver you dip into the water when the tides are low. Coming back up when she inhales, move along the edge of the ocean that is defined by the rib cage and the pelvis. After the dive, gently move the water in a circular motion with your happy clockwise circles. Your slow, gentle, connective movement guides her mind and body to a state of bliss.

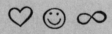

Trick of the Trade

Mother and Child Hand Technique

When one of your hands is working on your partner, the other hand is either active or passive. It feels good when the passive hand is in contact with the body, offering a nurturing presence, and knowing where your hands are is comforting to the receiver.

Align your right hand on her right waistline with your middle finger pointing to her belly button and left hand resting in front of the right hand. Together they form a belt. Now you are going to make some waves by rolling your hands across her belly starting with right heel, palm, fingers to left heel, palm,

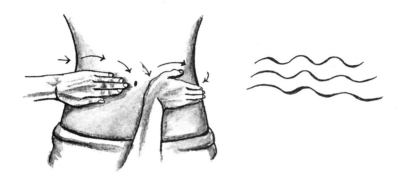

and fingers, then back to right heel where you started. Make more waves with your hands and slowly come to a still point, then go back to making circles. Transition to stand next to her hip, look into her face, and place your hands on each side of her belly button to create a butterfly. Reach both hands toward her

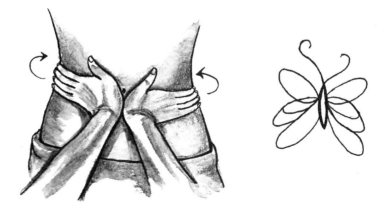

back, lifting her up, and let her gently back down on the table, your fingers following the belt and meeting at the belly button. Again, wrap your hands around her waist reaching her back, pulling her toward you, and then gently release, your fingers tracing her waistline and arriving at the belly button palms facing each other. Remember, third time's a charm, so repeat it one more time for good luck. Keep your palms together and glide the pinky side of your hands from her belly up to her chest as if you were swimming. Upon reaching the pectoralis muscle, separate your hands, place your right palm on her left pectoralis and your left hand on her right pectoralis, push down, and glide out when she exhales. From her pecs, move bilaterally to her shoulders and swim down her arms, reaching her fingertips, and swim off her body.

While I was studying Thai massage at the International Training Massage School (ITM) in Chiang Mai, my instructor told a funny story about using belly massage for constipation and diarrhea.

"You have been sitting on the toilet for about twenty minutes reading a book but nothing happened," he said matter-of-factly. "So you grab your smartphone to check emails and another ten minutes went by. Still no luck. All you need to do is press the pad of your palm toward your belly button and work on the whole belly this way and remember to do it clockwise. Pretty soon you will hear "plump!" and you can smile. But if you are having diarrhea, you should work counterclockwise instead."

Take a moment to shake out your hands and stretch. Undrape her right leg. Once you are ready, gather refreshed energy in your hands and reconnect with her body by moving from her right hip, down her leg, and to her toes. Going back up, hold her foot in your hands, making a "Foot Sandwich." Fingers tracing

the ankle, draw circles, moving
your hands on top of the leg,
and extending your thumbs out
to make a "U" shape. Place a
U on top of each leg to feel the
muscles under your thumbs and
fingers. Move your U toward the
knee and upon arrival turn your
body and your upper U to face
her right knee so you are making
a "( )" with both hands around
the knee for a "Knee Sandwich."

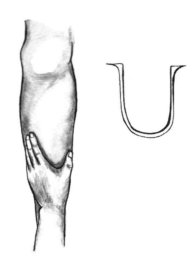

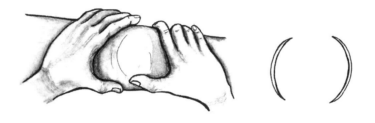

Grasping the tendon around the knee, make small, soothing
circles. Then your left and right hands take turns doing cross-fiber work on the thigh (quadriceps femoris). Position your hands
facing the same direction on each side of the thigh and work
across the muscle at the same time until you cover the whole
area. Turn your body around to face her head, then drag and pull
your hands down while you are moving back down to her toes.
Go up her leg again with the U hands, brush over the knee, and
join your fingers together in prayer position. Continue moving up onto the thigh. Separate your hands before arriving at
the hip, keeping the right hand on the thigh while the left hand,
with palm facing up, moves under her waist. Reach as far up her

back as you can, then scoop down her back and move back to the
hip. Place your left hand under the thigh to be directly beneath
the right hand to make the "Thigh Sandwich," hands moving
toward the knee. Once there, your right hand moves under the

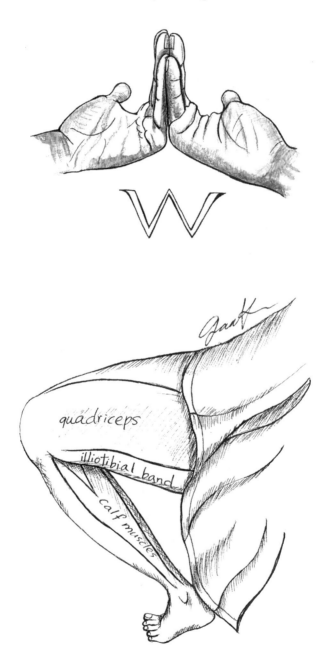

left hand to bend the knee slightly and pull the thigh toward you, stretching her hip. With both hands under the leg, interlace your fingers to make "W's." Your fingers should be in contact with her calf as you move toward the foot using the weight of her leg to provide the pressure. Now, with her heel supported in your left hand and your right hand holding her foot, lean back, shifting your weight to your back foot, to stretch her leg. Going up the leg for the third time, slightly increase the pressure. Once arriving at the thigh, place your left hand on the outside of the thigh (ITB). Use your forearm for anchoring while going up this large muscle group. Your left hand is in control of which part of her thigh to work on, so you take the time to explore different angles, possibilities and scenarios. Once satisfied, your left hand moves on to her back, making a connection that reminds her that the body is *one* entity: front, back, up, down and the sides. Make a Thigh Sandwich and move down to the knee, then use a "W" hand position to work on the calf while your thumbs are on either side of the shin. Then step back and give the leg a nice tug.

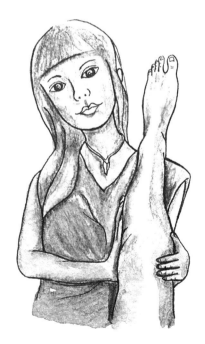

The space between her knee and the table is like the eye of a needle and you are threading the sheet corner from inside of her knee to the outside. Like making origami, you fold a corner of the sheet back onto her thigh, your left hand securing the sheet. Standing with your left leg in front of your right in a lunge position, place your right hand under her right ankle and slide it up her calf toward her knee so that her leg is supported by your forearm. Ground yourself and move from your core as you lift the leg up by bending her knee, bringing it toward her, and resting her foot on your right shoul-

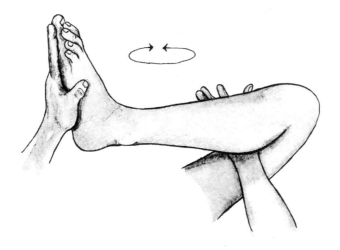

der. Place your right hand above her knee inside the thigh to keep the leg from flapping around. You are going to open up her hip joint by taking her leg out for a spin. You accomplish this effect by turning your whole body clockwise and counterclockwise. Just like in a trance music party, you are moving with the rhythm. Once the hip is nicely opened, bring the knee toward her right shoulder until you feel muscle resistance. Press your left hand on her hamstring behind the knee and with your right hand lift up her

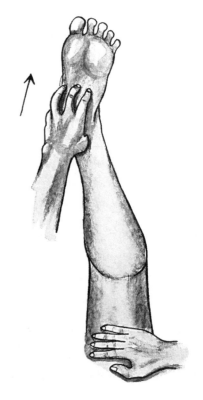

heel. Press and lift until you cover the whole hamstring. With the knee still bent, gently place her right foot across the body to land on the outside of her left knee. Press your left hand on her foot for anchoring, then walk around the table to stand on her left side, facing her head. Check in with her on the stretch and adjust the draping so she is properly covered – no wardrobe mal-function here. Place your

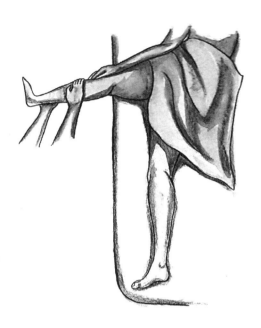

left hand on her lower back while your right hand supports her right knee and bring her back toward you, pushing her knee to-ward the table. This motion encourages her to lie on her left side. Rest her bent knee on your right hip, "hooked" on you. Your body is supporting her body and you move together as one. Both

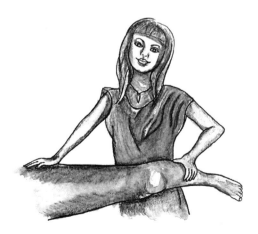

your hands are free to venture on her back, sacrum and gluteus, then simply turn yourself around to face her foot, putting her quads, ITB and calf under your fingertips. Explore these areas and slowly extend her bent knee to stretch her hamstring. This is a good place to pause and check in with her and yourself. Is she comfortable? Is your body aligned? Are you moving from your core?

Support her right leg with both hands and slowly walk around the table to bring her leg back to her right side. Gently bending her knee again, place her right foot on the table and guide her knee toward the right side of her body, opening up the adductor muscles in the inside of her thigh. You see that her knee is unable to rest all the way on the table so you add a little pillow for support. Start with soft hands to warm up the muscle, then increase the pressure by using the meaty part of your forearm. Slowly lift

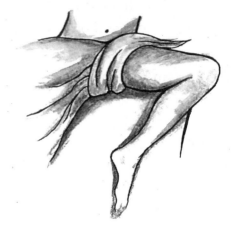

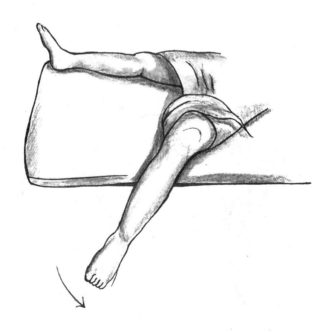

the knee so the leg is aligned with the hip and rest the right sole back on the table. Your left hand is providing support behind the knee, extending the leg, and your right hand is on her Achilles tendon. Swing her leg out to stretch the inside of the thigh further. Noting that her hip and the opposite leg are moving along, you check in on her comfort level and pay particular attention to her left foot: Once it is vertical to the table, you can stop and hold the stretch. Swing the leg back on the table, adjust the draping as needed, and gently give the leg a tug.

Attentively uncover the right side of her body and leave the hand towel covering her chest. Standing by her right foot in the lunge position, make the Foot Sandwich with your hands and move up the leg with U-shaped hands. Use your right forearm to continue to her thigh while your left hand, on the ITB, guides the angle of contact. Upon reaching her hip slowly dance your forearm back toward you and let your hand take the lead to gently glide onto her abdomen while your left hand moves to her lower back. The right hand continues up to her chest and the pectoralis muscle, then the left hand slides out from under her back to touch her ear and neck, then moves under her shoulder blade. Your right and left hands are embracing her shoulder, making a nice yummy "Shoulder Sandwich." As both hands move down the arm at the same time, your right elbow makes contact with her ITB. Your hands exit her fingers but your right elbow remains connected to her thigh. The elbow continues to move diagonally from the ITB to the inner thigh, bringing your hands to her knee. Reach behind the knee to form the W's with your fingers and continue down to the ankle. Rotate the ankle toward the arch, tug on the leg, and wiggle and pull on each toe. Turn your body so you are facing away from her head, pick up her right foot, and then slide your bended left leg under it.

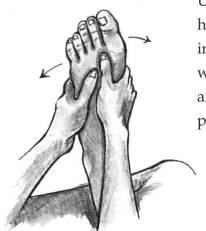

Use the heel of your hands to rub her Achilles tendon, like a washing machine agitator. Her sole is within reach of your fingertips and you soothe her by gently pulling and stretching.

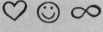

Trick of the Trade

Proper Draping

Gently pull and tug the sheet when draping the torso. For covering the limbs, grab the sheet corner and pull it from inside the limb toward the outside. When undraping, directly pulling the sheet can feel uncomfortable to the sensitive skin. So instead, gently lift the body and pull the sheet away.

You are holding her feet in your hands with alternating pressure, rocking your body left to right to left and using this opportunity to rotate your neck, shoulder and hip. Repeat the rocking with the rhythm ending on her left foot. Move the drape to uncover her left leg, then apply lotion from her toes up to her hip and back down to her toes. Be alert to any tension that stands out. Start with Foot Sandwich as the appetizer, moving to U-shaped hands for holding the soup, and then serve up a Knee Sandwich as the entree. Next, mix salad dressing with your hands on her thigh, then help the hostess make noodles by dragging your hands down from her thigh to her toes. You enjoyed your meal and decide to go back for second helpings. You have the Foot Sandwich and your U-shaped bowl for the soup, then lace your fingers in prayer position to give thanks for this delicious meal. Your left hand reaches behind her back to gather some fallen bread crumbs and you are ready for the Thigh Sandwich. You notice you are getting thirsty, so you reach back her leg to get a drink of water by making a W with your fingers. Now you are getting a little full, so you hold onto her foot, lean back, and stretch. That was a great dining experience – going back for the third time was an easy decision. The Foot Sandwich and soup are already there waiting for you. Wanting to show your appreciation, you help your hostess straighten out some knots on the tablecloth that is lying across her thigh, using your left forearm while your right hand, on her ITB, keeps the tablecloth steady. You remember to reach back and scoop up the fallen bread crumbs. She thanks you by giving you a Thigh Sandwich and some water for the trip home.

You are having such a wonderful time, so go back for another visit. She needs some help in the kitchen, so without hesitation you properly drape the working area, threading the sheet under her knee then lifting up the large spatula (her leg) and resting it on your shoulder. You're now ready to mix a giant bowl of cookie dough. With your legs grounded and moving from your core, turn the spatula both clockwise and counterclockwise. Then, using your right hand as cookie cutter, press down on her hamstring and lift up her heel with your left hand, yielding three palm-size cookies. Now you are going to help her make some taffy! The secret to good taffy is stretching, pulling and twisting. Stretch her leg across her body to give the left side a nice twist, then follow up the stretch by walking to stand close to her right leg, where you hook her bent knee on your waist. You are now ready to do some pulling, beginning with the space on her back and moving on to the gluteal area. Then turn around to do more stretching on the quads, ITB and calf muscles. Unbend her knee to stretch her hamstring and gently return her leg to her left side. Follow by bending her left knee then resting her foot on the table. Open the oven door by gently bringing her bended knee to her left and resting it on the table; you are now able to access her inner thigh (adductor muscles). Carefully slide in the cookie sheet, first with your palm and then forearm. Once the cookies are done baking you close the oven door and return her left leg back to the table. Align her left leg with the hip and swing the whole leg out to stretch inside her leg until you feel the resistance, then swing the leg back on the table, this time stretching her leg toward her feet.

Open the sheet to uncover the left side of her body and take a look and see the connection from the top of her shoulder to the bottom of her foot. With your nurturing hands contact her foot, embrace it, and move up this leg with a familiar touch. Remember to reach back and pay attention to her back with your right hand while your left hand is slithering up her belly

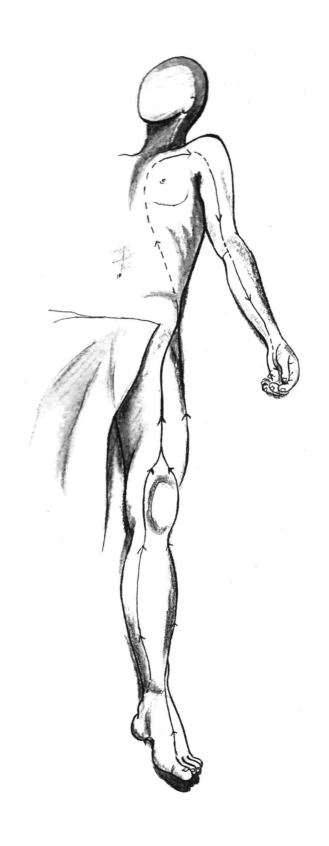

like a snake. With both hands, embrace the shoulder and glide down the arm while your left elbow starts to make contact with her ITB. Your hands are moving down the fingers and your left elbow is moving toward inside her knee. Together your hands arrive briefly at her calf, then gracefully come to her foot, where you hold, pause and stretch.

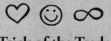

Trick of the Trade

Focusing

It takes astute observation to notice a client's muscle tension, and it is definitely important to know what is "wrong" with him. But when a client asks me, "Do I have the worst shoulder you have ever seen?" instead of agreeing or disagreeing, I shift the focus to what is "right." I talk about how well his body is working and ask what kind of change he would like for himself.

This gives my client a chance to acknowledge all the wonderful workings in his body and empowers him to work toward positive change. "Your focus determines your reality," says Qui-Gon Jinn to Obi Wan. To focus on all the "wrongs" makes progress an endless uphill battle-there will constantly be something to "fix." Focusing positively on how we would like to improve and grow so things can function even better is a more compassionate way to view our body.

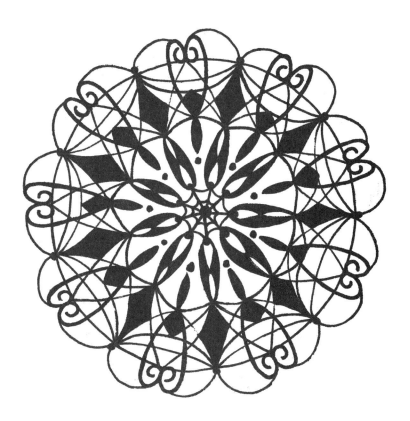

9

'I have just three things to teach:
simplicity, patience, compassion.
These three are your greatest treasures.'
~ Lao Tzu~

Wow, we have come a long way from our humble beginning, from noticing and working with our own breath to extending that awareness to our partner, coupled with various massage techniques. (Let's hope by now you are falling fast asleep – that is, if you are the one who is receiving a massage.)

In the beginning of the book we talked about how the body is one entity, not a collection of separate quadrants. To see the body as composed of "parts" sounds like we're talking about Frankenstein's monster; leave the horror to Mary Shelley and Hollywood and embrace the beautiful on our massage table. And be patient: The flow of massage comes with practice; it is common to find yourself thinking about the next move. "I just finished warming up my hands and now my partner is covered with this fancy vegan organic lotion," you think to yourself. "Should I go to her shoulder or her lower back?" I say go wherever feels right and ask for her feedback.

Scan, Focus and Act is the creative thinking process created by Matt and Gail Taylor that was introduced to me while working on the Web and graphic production team at KnOwhere Store eons ago. The same cerebral process works well for the intuitive touch. Intuitively, your hands travel down her back and you *scan* the body and notice the muscles of her lower back feel more tense. So naturally you stay there, *focusing* to find out which side of the lower back can use more tender loving care. Define the area by looking for any sensation that stands out, such as restricted movement. When you glide your hands through an area, ask yourself, "Does it feel like I am driving over a speed bump?" Your *action* is to follow the muscle fiber direction to help lengthen it. The Scan, Focus and Act continues: While you are elongating the muscle, you are *scanning* to see if there is anything that stands out with that particular muscle. Maybe it feels like tiny rocks. Once you find the spot, *focus* your attention there and sync your breath with your partner's. Now your *action* is to stay on that area with your index and middle fingers. Wait until you feel the muscle start to soften. During the period of waiting, you are *scanning* to see if the area is indeed responding to your touch. Is it an apple or an orange? If it is pliant like an orange, that means keep on doing what you are doing until the tension releases. If it is hard like an apple, shift the gear to *focus*, really clear your head of any noise, and be mindful of what's happening under your fingertips. Be like Sherlock Holmes looking for clues – the answer to defeat the knot is consistency and ingenuity. Your *action* toward a hard apple is to be flexible. When one massage technique does not work, try a different one. For example, maybe you have been favoring a cross-fiber move; it makes you feel tough by confronting the knot directly. You remember to check in with your partner on the pressure and it is good. However, after working at it for more than two minutes, the tension remains. You decide to use anchor-and-pull technique by pressing on the knot and moving her leg slowly in the opposite direction to create more space for the lower back. By doing this you are combining pressure, lengthening, and stretching all at the same time. Her lower back finally loosens up. After the intensive workout you gently go over the whole lower back with a soothing, nurturing touch.

Another component of ingenuity is knowing when to leave an area alone. Yes, leaving it alone is just as important as continuing to work. Massage really is about simplicity, patience and compassion. Sometimes you need to give the knot a chance to conform by giving it space and time. It's like putting together the 2,000-piece Van Gogh's *Starry Night* puzzle: If a piece stumps you, you can't get mad and throw it into the trash, or keep on forcing it to fit where it does not. That would certainly not help the situation. The sensible solution is to put together the pieces you know while keeping the shape of the mystery piece in mind, checking every once in a while to see if you've found the spot on the board that is your salvation. The lower back tension might be related to a hip misalignment, so the back is refusing to relax until the hip is taken care of. Or maybe a tight abdominal muscle is pulling on the lower back. A weak ankle might even be the cause. Although far from the lower back, that ankle could be compromising the body balance and in turn causing the lower back tension. Not your usual suspect, but like they say, it's the quiet ones you have to watch. When you realize that the possibilities are endless, the method of trying to beat the muscle into submission suddenly seems barbaric.

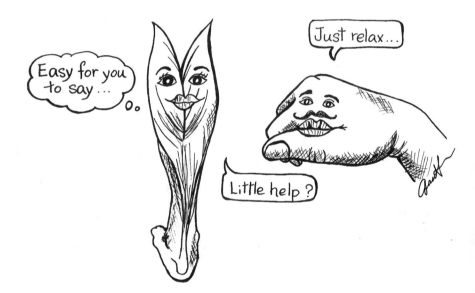

About three months ago, one of my clients dislocated his pinky as a result of saving his toddler from diving over the edge of the crib. Even though he injured only the pinky, the pain was causing his whole body to tense up, as if someone had turned on an alert button, and now his whole body was on constant fight, flight and freeze response. While my client's story was still fresh in my mind, I signed up for John Barnes' Myofascial Release and Unwinding workshop in San Francisco. In John's intensive workshop, he continually reminded therapists to think of the body as a whole system without up, down, left, right, front or back, because fascia, the connective tissue throughout our whole body, is one continuum and does not care about our linear view of the world. Once again, this confirms the theory that treating the symptom is not enough for healing unless we find the cause of the pain. There is a poster of an iceberg hanging in my chiropractor Dr. Stewart's treatment room. The part of the iceberg that is above sea level says, "Symptoms are misleading." The part of the iceberg that is under the water is nine times the size and says, "We find the hidden cause." And when I lie face up on the treatment table there is a secret note posted on the ceiling. "Trust and come into your senses." Ah, Dr. Stewart, how very wise you are.

Since we are talking about logic and intuition, I am tempted to ask, "Would you fix a smartphone with a hammer?" Before you answer, know that this is not a trick question. If the only tool you have is a hammer, the probability of you using it increases greatly. Now, I admit a smartphone can be pretty awesome. Mine remembers all my friends' numbers and birthdays, sends out alerts for important to-dos, corrects my spelling (although sometimes over-corrects, like the time I was meeting up with friends for dinner and I texted them, "I am parked next to the hot tub place," and my phone turned it into, "I am parked next to the horrible." What the duck!?) I also love the fact that I can play Tetris while listening to Gillian Welch. But before artificial intelligence overpowers and conquers the human race, and before we give robots massage, I stand firm on the belief that we are far more fascinating than metal-wrapped silicon that sends out and receives electrical signal of zeros and ones. I declare that the body is far more sophisticated than a phone. Take the ears. "Rolls of pleasure roll sound waves down the auditory canal to the eardrum, causing it to vibrate," Robert Ornstein writes in *Evolution of Consciousness*. "The vibration of the eardrum causes the three bones of the middle ear (ossicles) to vibrate.... Their vibrations match the original signal in frequency but are of greater amplitude (twenty-five times greater). The pressure of that amplification forces the waves into the inner ear, where they are transduced into electrical energy in the nerve cells. And in the brain we hear Mozart, the sound of waterfalls, poetry, and the complaints of our neighbors." You probably remember that piece of information from biology class, and yet it is still amazingly profound to be reminded of the intricate engineering of you and me.

So along with not taking a hammer to our smartphone, I believe we have established that we should avoid forceful intention while working with our partner and instead utilize different tools when necessary. When you feel your hands are getting tired or sore, switch to fists, forearms, elbows or knees instead. Again, listen to your body, check in with your feet. Are they grounded? Are your knees slightly bent? Is your spine settled comfortably on top of your pelvis? Where are your shoulders and neck? Are they relaxed? Connect with yourself and with your partner. E.M. Forster says, "Only Connect." He is right.

Slowly you are coming to the end of the massage session, and the end is as important as the beginning, requiring the same presence, love and gratitude. You are standing on the left

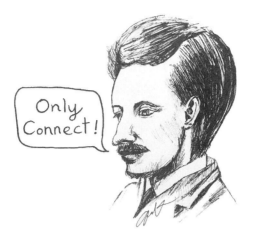

Only Connect!

side of your partner with your right hand cradling his neck and your left middle finger resting on top of his head. If you draw a line from the uppermost point of his ears toward the center of his head, you will land right on Governing Vessel 20 - Hundred Meetings. In acupressure this point facilitates calmness. Light pressure is all you need. Breathe with him. Stay there until his body is ready for you to move on. How do you know when that is? When is the "right moment"? Often you can hear or see your partner's breath deepen and you can feel the pulse slow down. Patiently wait until he exhales, then place your left finger on his third eye. Take a couple of mindful breaths and place your left hand on his chest. Let your palm rest on his sternum with your index and thumb beneath his collarbone. Travel to a peaceful place in your mind while connecting with your partner. Bring your right hand from under his neck to join your left hand, and let them both melt in this wonderful sensation of stillness. Your hands take turns brushing down his sternum. Rest your right hand on his stomach and left hand below his belly button. Wait a couple of breaths, then on the next inhalation raise your hands and touch his left shoulder with your right hand and his right hip with your left hand.

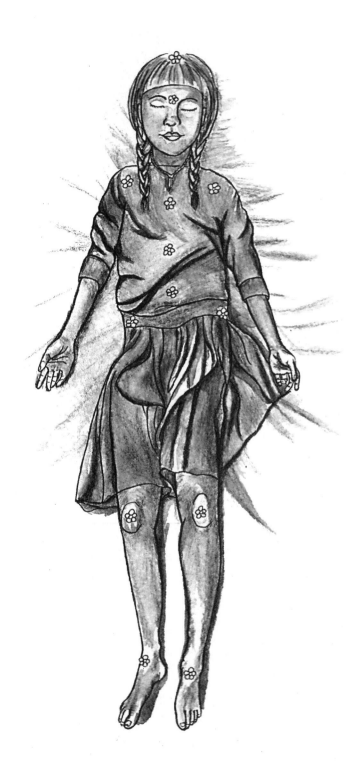

This technique is borrowed from polarity therapy, which is based on the body's complex energetic system. To simplify the idea, the top right side of our body is positively charged and left bottom side is negatively charged. By placing your hands on your partner, you are facilitating the balance of his vital life force. Place your right hand on his left shoulder and your left hand on his right hip. Once you feel there is a release, move your right hand to his left shoulder and left hand to his right hip. This criss-crossing hand movement keeps you from falling asleep. Continually move the energy down, your right hand on his right hip and left hand on his left knee. Switch: your right hand on his left hip and left hand on his right knee. Then – you guessed it! – your right hand goes to his left knee and left hand to his right ankle. When you are both ready, your right hand is now on his right knee and left hand on his left ankle. Now rest both your hands on his feet, then use thumb pressure to trace five lines from the heels toward each toe. Silently or audibly speak, chant or sing your blessing to your partner.

During one monthlong Esalen Massage training, I was fortunate to receive a massage session at the bathhouse perched on a cliff overlooking the Pacific. The sound of the waves pounding the Big Sur coast was both intense and soothing. The massage took me on a journey to my subconscious. It was a dreamlike world where I was a child, an adolescent and an adult all at the same time. Time progression was folded like an accordion, each part of me acquainted with the other me's. A song brought me back to this reality, and once I gained consciousness I was back in the bathhouse. My massage therapist was singing softly while ending the session. *"The universe is full of magical things, patiently waiting for our wits to grow sharper."* – *Eden Phillpotts*. I felt peaceful and loved and was reminded of all the goodness that

surrounds me. I seldom practice audible blessing in my work at
Google. Now, sharing this experience with you encourages me
to be brave and incorporate my voice as part of the healing tool.
Give it a try and see for yourself.

Finally, ask your partner to lie on his side, which encourages deeper relaxation. The fetal position reminds the body it
is safe. Wrap his body from head to toe tightly, as if you were
swaddling a baby. Brush your hands gently from the top of his
head and spread your index and middle fingers so they are in
contact with each side of the spine, and travel all the way down
to the sacrum for three minutes. This technique is called "nerve
stroke," from Carole Osborne's class, and helps to calm the ner-

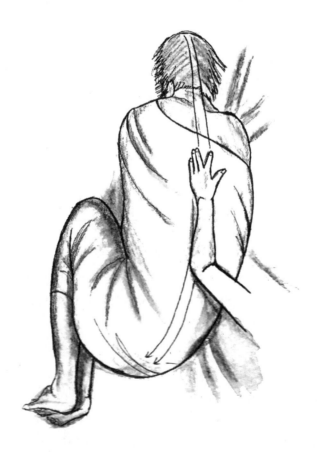

vous system. Slowly move your hands off his body, breathe, and move energetically off your partner. Breathe, ground yourself, shake your hands, shake your body, breathe and stretch your hands above your head. Stand on your tippy toes like you are catching monarchs. Breathe and let the positive energy, happy thoughts and love come into you. Breathe, stretch forward from your hip like you are picking e.e. cummings' burning flowers. Sink your hands on the ground, breathe, let all the negative energy, regret, grief, fear and shame be absorbed by the nurturing Mother Earth. Slowly rise like the morning sun, one vertebra at a time. Take your time. You are standing with intention and moving with purpose.

The journey of massage turns out to be a journey of self-discovery. There is no single, absolute way that each of us has to follow. We create our own path. The self is complex, composed of many intricate layers of tangible physical form and the intangible emotional formless form. Both are ever-changing, and no

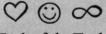

Trick of the Trade

Side-lying and Pregnancy Masage

Besides lying face up or face down on the massage table, your partner can also lie on her side. Side-lying is not only for the pregnant — it might be the only comfortable position for those using life-support devices and people with sinus issues.

There are many schools of thought on if and when a pregnant woman is able to receive massage. The rule of thumb is every pregnancy is different, so always check with your physician. For pregnancy massage, the intention is not deep but nurturing work, so gentle movement goes a long way. You will need two standard pillows, a body pillow and several other small pillows for support. When she is lying on her side with a standard pillow under her head, let her hug the body pillow with lower leg straightened and the top leg bent, draped over the body pillow. Check to see if her hip, knee and foot are aligned. Elevate the ankle so it is above the rest of the body if there are signs of water retention.

The following acupressure points are contraindicated in pregnancy:
• Gallbladder 21- Shoulder Well is on the shoulder directly above the nipples.
• Large Intestine 4 - Tiger's Mouth is on the fleshy spot between thumb and index finger.
• Kidney 1 - Bubbling Spring is on the sole; if you draw lines from the big, second and third toe they would meet at the point.
• Kidney 6 - Shining Sea is on the inside of the foot, directly below the middle of the ankle bone.
• Spleen 6 - Three Yin Intersection is on the inside of the leg the length of receiver's index finger above the ankle.
• Urinary Bladder 60 - Kunlun Mountains is in the depression between the outside ankle and Achilles tendon.
• Urinary Bladder 67 - Reaching Yin is on the outside of the small toe.

matter which point you happen to come across, know that point is connected to several other points. "Tug on anything at all and you'll find it connected to everything else in the universe," John Muir wrote. The self is fluid and has the ability to heal, transform and renew, if provided with nurturing touch and space. The self is a creature of habit and has the tendency of repeating – doing, thinking and being. I was in a Gestalt workshop hosted by Christine Price in Aptos, and one participant explained she had become friends with her right shoulder pain. She was afraid to let it go, because she might just float away without it. Her fear was real. I saw it in her eyes, the fear of being painless, the fear of being free from her burden. It sounded ridiculous. How could anyone be in love with their pain and suffering? Maybe she was feeling apprehension of something new, the not knowing? As she spoke, I saw an image of heavy broken pieces that longed for cohesion, a synchrony of self. The lightness of being and yet the lack of nurturing was restricting her from trusting herself to reach that wholeness. Oftentimes, the only person stopping us from attaining that harmony is our own self. When we reach into ourselves and reach out to others from a point of compassion, we are acknowledging that everything good in us echoes everything that is good in others. Embody the meaning of Namaste.

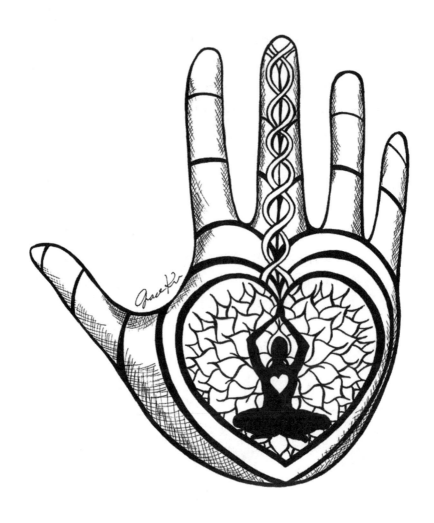

THREE • IMAGES

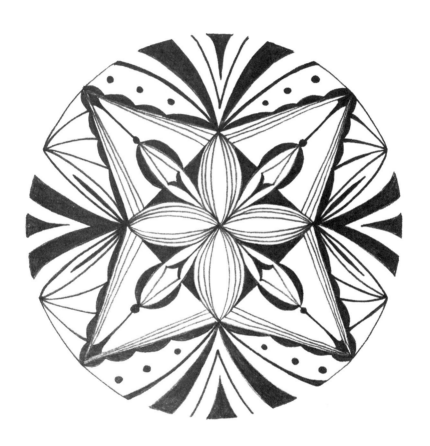

Yay! Now all the massage illustrations are at your fingertips with descriptions of techniques in back! This section is for visual learners like myself. Please feel free to use them to help you memorize the massage moves and even create your very own massage flow. You can also ask your partner to pick a couple of them randomly and practice on each other. So dim the lights, put on some soothing music and start your own magic.

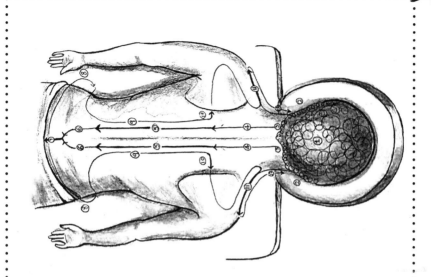

One Body Massage

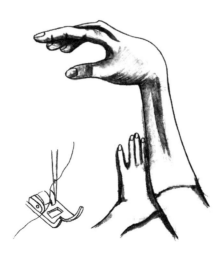

One Body Massage

1. head

2. base of scalp

3.–6. neck to back

7. sacrum

8. top of glutes, fingers grabbing hip

9. hands moving from hip to scapulae

10. hands pushing scapulae toward ears

11. hands pushing down shoulders

12. back to base of scalp

Slide your right elbow into the "L" and travel up his back on the erector spinae muscle group right next to the spine.

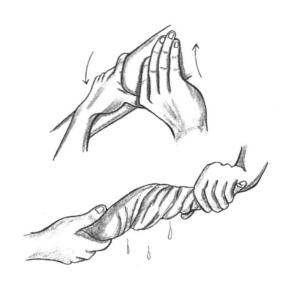

One Body Massage

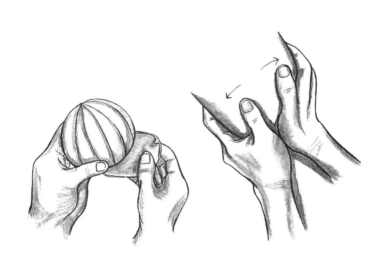

One Body Massage

Like wringing water off a wet towel, you wring the deltoid, triceps and biceps muscles.

Once you reach the forearm, you grasp in the middle of the forearm muscles and pull them away from each other to create the stretch, like opening up an orange.

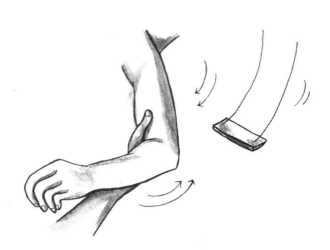

One Body Massage

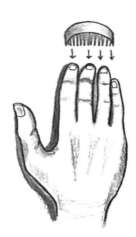

One Body Massage

With your left palm facing up, reach for his elbow and rest his left arm on your forearm. This way you are providing complete support and have great control of his arm. Stretch his triceps while his elbow is bent and straighten the arm to stretch the biceps, then go up to his deltoid.

Bend his elbow again to place your right fingers next to the spine. Start combing the muscles with your fingers from spine to shoulder blade, all the while swinging his arm from his left to right.

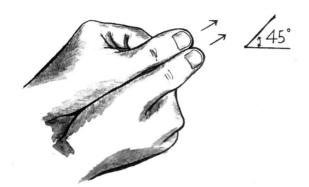

One Body Massage

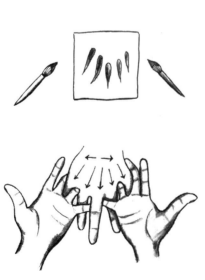

One Body Massage

With your left and right thumbs sitting side by side, lengthen the muscle from spine to shoulder blade at a forty-five-degree angle. You are like an artist sculpting a beautiful wing for an angel.

Now, with both your palms facing up, lace your right pinky between his mid and ring finger while your right ring finger slides between his index and thumb. Your left pinky is in between his mid and ring finger while your left ring finger is in between his ring and pinky. Your fingers are like the wooden frame, stretching and opening up space in his palm, which is like the canvas. Your thumbs are the brushes that are going to paint on the canvas.

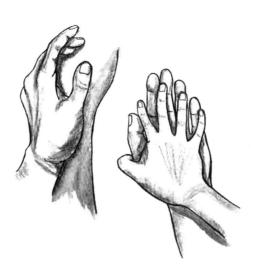

One Body Massage

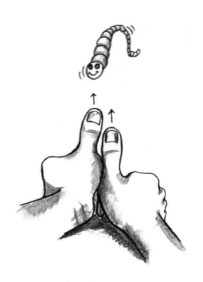

One Body Massage

Turn yourself around so you are facing his feet. As your left elbow goes down toward his lower back, your right hand is on his shoulder and glides toward his hand. Like two cars driving on different roads at different speeds but arriving at their destination at the same time.

Your intention is to lengthen this muscle, quadratus lumborum (QL), by pushing the QL down toward the top of the pelvis. After warming up the QL, you go deeper by using rhythmic movement one thumb at a time, moving forward little by little. This movement generates from your hip.

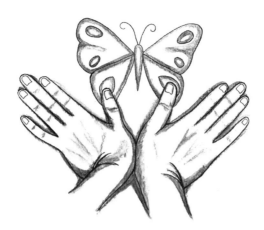

One Body Massage

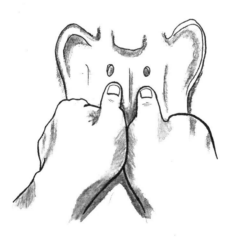

One Body Massage

With your palms facing down side by side like a butterfly, push the sacrum toward her feet, stretching and opening up this area.

Now go deeper at more specific points by using your thumbs. Applying shiatsu technique, sink your thumbs in between the first and second fused verte-brae when she exhales. Let go of the thumb pressure when she inhales and repeat this process a couple more times till you cover her whole sacrum.

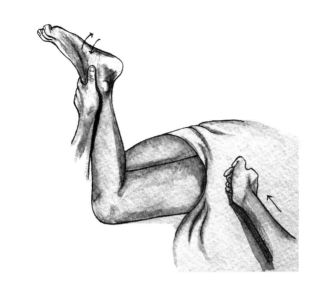

One Body Massage

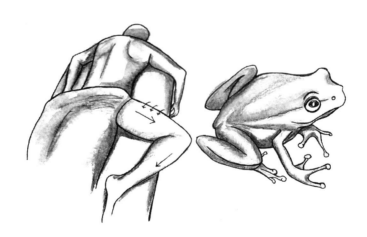

One Body Massage

Moving your left hand to support her foot, keep the knee bent ninety degrees and make a soft fist on her gluteus with your right hand. Bring her foot toward you and push down on her gluteus at the same time. This stretches her piriformis and provides a deep opening for her hip.

You are standing at her feet, facing her. With your right hand under her knee and your left hand on her foot, lift her right leg by resting her foot on your shoulder. Now gently bring her knee out to the right and rest the leg on the table. The frog position gives you easy access to her ITB, part of her quads, and the muscle outside the shin (tibialis anterior), and at the same time stretches her inner thigh, warming up the muscles from her foot to ITB and the side of her hip.

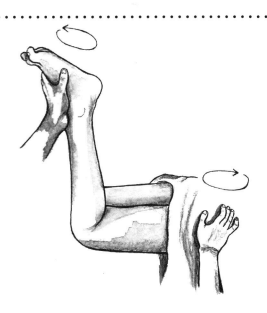

One Body Massage

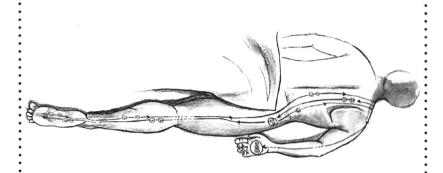

One Body Massage

With the knee still bent, move your right palm onto her gluteus, your fingers in contact with her sacrum, and rotate her foot counterclockwise. You're pressing down on her gluteus and moving your right hand clockwise at the same time.

Your right hand is leading and left forearm is following. Glide back from her arm to shoulder, turn to face her foot, your right forearm gliding down her back while your left hand moves down her arm at the same time. Forearm and hand meet together at the gluteus and move down the leg together. The third time is just the same, except when the forearm and hand meet at the gluteal, the right hand goes back up to the shoulder and the left hand goes down the leg.

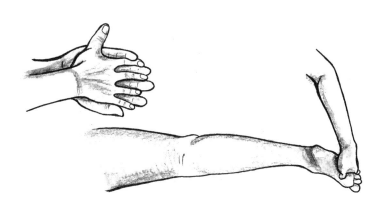

One Body Massage

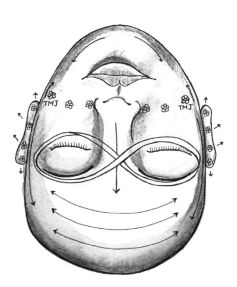

One Body Massage

Your right hand arrives at her hand and your left hand reaches her foot at the same time.

"Infinity Glasses" Trace under the right eye orbit, moving up across the nose ridge and tracing above the left eyebrow ridge, then traveling down to the left temporal lobe, going under the left eye orbit across the nose ridge, curving above the right eyebrow ridge, and arriving back where you started. Massage the right temple in a circular motion, then bring the left fingers into the rhythm on the opposite temple. Repeat the Infinity Glasses starting from the left temple.

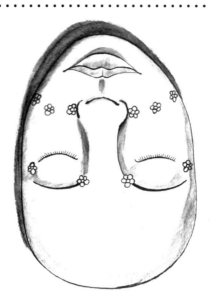

One Body Massage

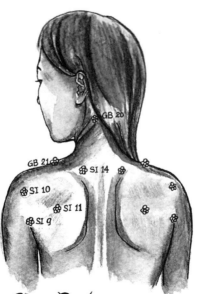

One Body Massage

174

"Beauty Mask" Land your thumbs on his third eye and slide right to where the eyebrows begin, index fingers on both sides of the nose, middle fingers underneath the middle of the cheek bone, ring fingers bent to place on the temples, pinkies reaching for the TMJs.

SI 9: above the armpit crease

SI 10: four fingers above SI9 and sink in

SI 11: middle of the shoulder blade

SI 14: above the inner edge of the shoulder blade on the line lateral to the lower border of spinous process of the 1st thoracic vertebra.

GB 21: along middle top of the trapezius

GB 20: at the base of the skull in the hollows

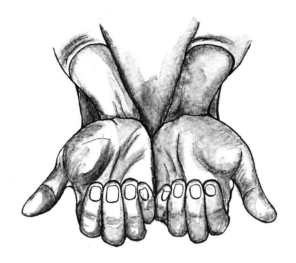

One Body Massage

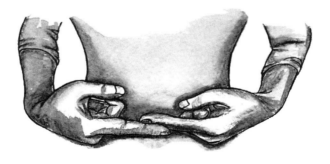

One Body Massage

CV4: Slide your hands to the base of the skull and lift up his head so your fingertips are supporting the weight. Your fingertips are in contact with deep neck muscles

Bring your hands underneath the neck with index fingers contacting the cervical vertebrae and the rest of the hands there to support the weight of the neck. Each index finger takes turns leading the stretch. One cervical vertebra at a time, moving all the way up to the base of the skull. It is like your index fingers are playing hide-and-seek.

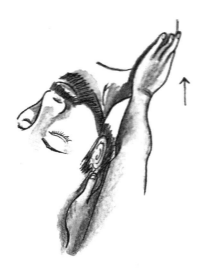

One Body Massage

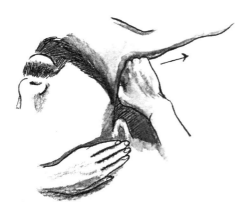

One Body Massage

Lift his head off the table with both your hands and bring his head toward his left shoulder, keeping his nose pointing to the sky until you reach a point of resistance.

Then rest his head back on the table and with your right hand supporting the head like an anchor, push down on his right shoulder with your left palm. You are crossing your arms to stretch his trapezius.

Make a soft fist with your right hand, palm facing down – as if you were holding an egg – and trace the muscle from the base of the neck back to the shoulder.

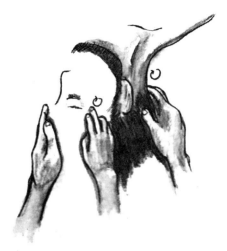

One Body Massage

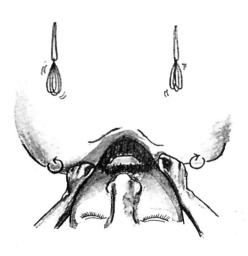

One Body Massage

Turn his head to the left, so his nose is now facing left then stretch. Make happy circles from the base of his head (occiput), up behind his ears, circling on his temple and back down to the occiput.

With two egg-holding fists you will turn the right wrist clockwise and the left one counterclockwise at the same time, imagining you are making scrambled eggs. You are beating the eggs starting from the base of the neck toward the shoulder and back to the neck, and you are repeating the wrist rotation until everything is nice and fluffy.

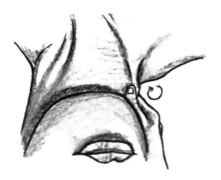

One Body Massage

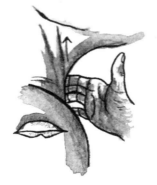

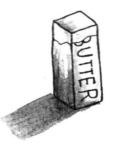

One Body Massage

Turn his head so his nose is now pointing to the right. Ask him to lift up his head slightly so you can see his sternocleidomastoid (SCM) muscle, popping out to say hello. With his head still supported in your left hand, turn to the right and grab his SCM with your thumb and index finger; with this motion, like twisting to close a bottle cap, you are working the whole SCM.

Keep his head turned to the right. Find his scalenes by sliding your thumb right behind the SCM. Feel the scalenes with your fingers and trace the muscles from the base of the head (occiput) toward the collabone (clavicle). You want to slowly warm the region.

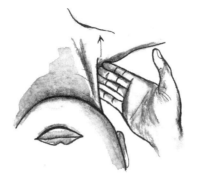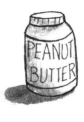

One Body Massage

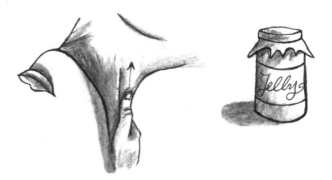

One Body Massage

Align his head with the rest of his body and spread the peanut butter on the scalenes until it is nicely covered.

Turn his head by pointing his nose to the left and cover the scalenes with jelly.

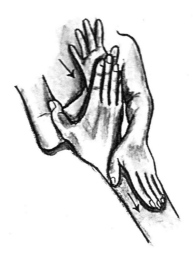

One Body Massage

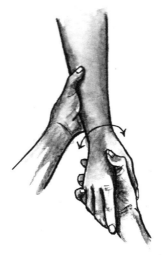

One Body Massage

186

Keeping his hand on the table with palm facing down, each time you lift his fingers to reveal his palm with your right hand, your left hand will press down on his forearm and push up toward his elbow to create a "pumping" motion. Lift and glide until his whole forearm gets a good workout.

Holding his hand in the handshake position, squeeze the forearm with your left thumb, index and middle fingers while turning his wrist to increase the sensation.

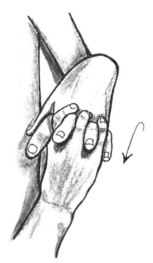

One Body Massage

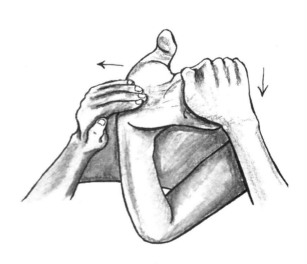

One Body Massage

Lace your fingers with his palm facing yours and bring his elbow to ninety degrees. Brace his wrist with your left thumb and index finger and rotate the wrist. Dig your fingertips between his knuckles to stretch his fingers.

Rest his elbow on the table while your left hand stretches his fingers to keep the palm open, facing the sky, and your right fingertips comb the palm.

189

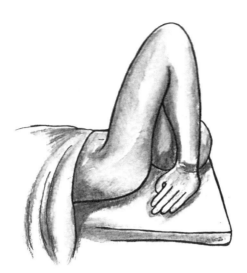

One Body Massage

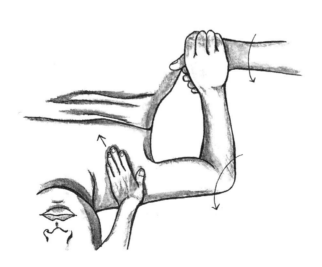

One Body Massage

Keep his palm open and tilt his elbow up to face the sky with help from your right hand so his palm is touching the table right by his head.

Holding his hand in arm-wrestle position, drop the elbow on the table so the forearm and elbow form a ninety degree angle. With his hand still in yours, turn to face his feet. Your left fingertips are getting ready to comb his pectoralis by finding the groove that is right next to the shoulder and right below the clavicle. Your left fingers are combing from groove to sternum while your right hand is stretching his hand toward his head.

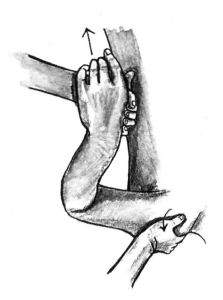

One Body Massage

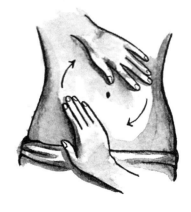

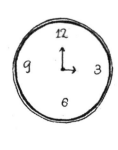

One Body Massage

With his hand still in yours, and the elbow and forearm still at ninety degrees, move to stand parallel to his shoulder. Your left hand is grabbing his deltoid. Bring his hand down toward his feet, while your left hand is pretending to peel the deltoid off his shoulder by grasping and pulling it towards his head.

Her inhalation is a cue to start drawing clockwise circles with your hands from small to large, using her belly button as the focal point.

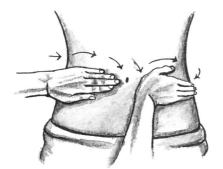

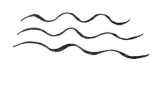

One Body Massage

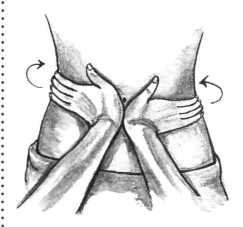

One Body Massage

194

Align your right hand on her right waistline with your middle finger pointing to her belly button and left hand resting in front of the right hand. Together they form a belt. Now you are going to make some waves by rolling your hands across her belly starting with right heel, palm, fingers to left heel, palm and fingers, then back to right heel where you started.

Transition to stand next to her hip and look into her face, place your hands on each side of her belly button to create a butterfly. Reach both hands toward her back, lifting her up, and let her gently back down on the table, your fingers following the belt and meeting at the belly button.

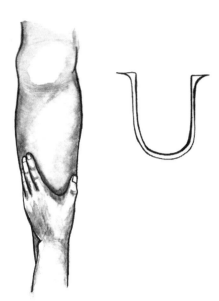

One Body Massage

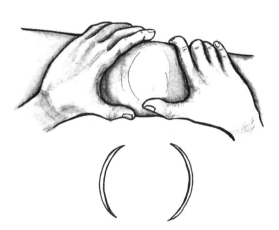

One Body Massage

Fingers tracing the ankle, draw circles, moving hands on top of the leg, extending thumbs out to make a "U" shape. Place a U on top of each leg to feel the muscles under your thumbs and fingers. Move your U toward the knee.

You are making a ( ) with both hands around the knee for a Knee Sandwich. Grasping the tendon around the knee, make small soothing circles.

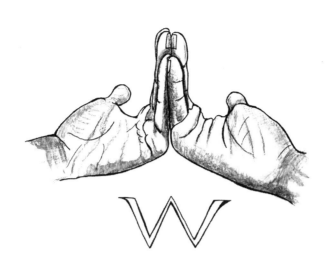

One Body Massage

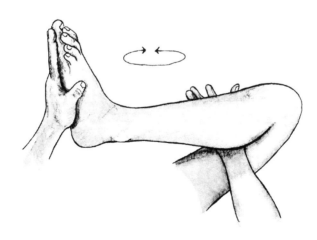

One Body Massage

198

Interlace your fingers to make "W's." Your fingers should be in contact with her calf as you move toward the foot using the weight of her leg to provide the pressure.

Place your right hand above her knee inside the thigh to keep the leg from flapping around. You are going to open up her hip joint by taking her leg out for a spin. You accomplish this effect by turning your whole body clockwise and counterclockwise.

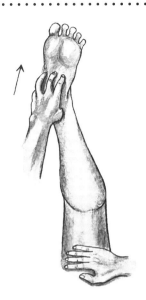

One Body Massage

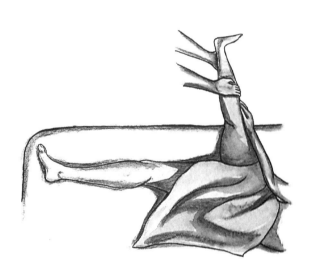

One Body Massage

Bring the knee toward her right shoulder until you feel muscle resistance. Press your left hand on her hamstring behind the knee and with your right hand lift up her heel. Press and lift until you cover the whole hamstring.

With the knee still bent, gently place her right foot across the body to land on the outside of her left knee. Press your left hand on her foot for anchoring, then walk around the table to stand on her left side, facing her head. Place your left hand on her lower back while your right hand supports her right knee and bring her back toward you, pushing her knee toward the table. This motion encourages her to lie on her left side.

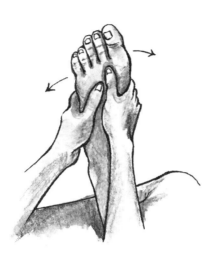

One Body Massage

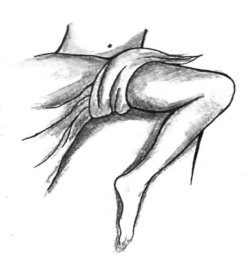

One Body Massage

Turn your body so you are facing away from her head, pick up her right foot, and then slide your bended left leg under it. Use the heel of your hands to rub her Achilles tendon, like a washing machine agitator. Her sole is within reach of your fingertips and you soothe her by gently pulling and stretching.

Gently bending her knee again, place her right foot on the table and guide her knee toward the right side of her body, opening up the adductor muscles in the inside of her thigh. Start with soft hands to warm up the muscle, then increase the pressure by using the meaty part of your forearm.

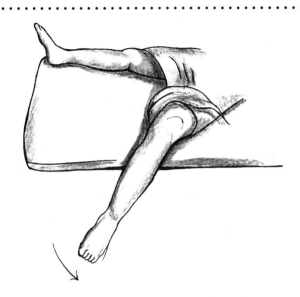

One Body Massage

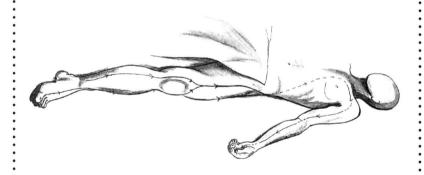

One Body Massage

Slowly lift the knee so the leg is aligned with the hip, and rest the right sole back on the table. Your left hand is providing support behind the knee, extending the leg, and your right hand is on her Achilles tendon. Swing her leg out to stretch the inside the thigh further. Noting that her hip and the opposite leg are moving along, you check in on her comfort level and pay particular attention to her left foot: Once it is vertical to the table, you can stop and hold the stretch.

Open the sheet to uncover the left side of her body, contact her foot, embrace it, and move up her leg with a familiar touch. Remember to reach back and pay attention to her back with your right hand while your left hand is slithering up her belly like a snake. With both hands, embrace the shoulder and glide down the arm while your left elbow starts to make contact with her ITB. Your hands are moving down the fingers and your left elbow moving toward inside her knee. Together your hands move to be in touch with her calf, then gracefully come to her foot.

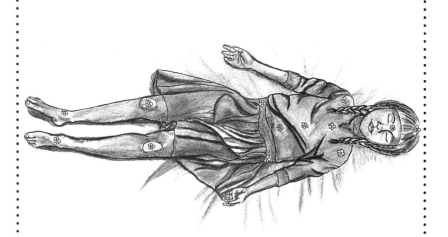

One Body Massage

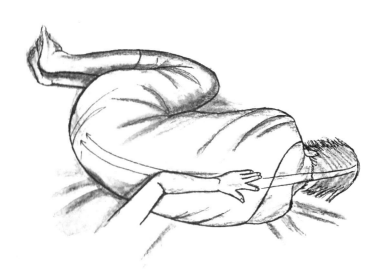

One Body Massage

You are standing on the left side of your partner with your right hand cradling his neck and your left middle finger resting on top of his head. Place your left finger on his third eye. Let your palm rest on his sternum with your index and thumb beneath his collarbone. Your left hand on his right shoulder and your right hand on his left hip. Your left hand on his right hip and right hand on his left knee. Switch: your right hand on his left hip and left hand on his right knee. Then your right hand goes to his left knee and left hand to his right ankle. Your left hand is now on his right knee and right hand on his left ankle. Rest both your hands on his feet.

The fetal position reminds the body it is safe. Wrap his body from head to toe tightly, as if you were swaddling a baby. Brush your hands gently from the top of his head and spread your index and middle fingers so they are in contact with each side of the spine, and travel all the way down to the sacrum for three minutes.

FOUR • ASPECTS

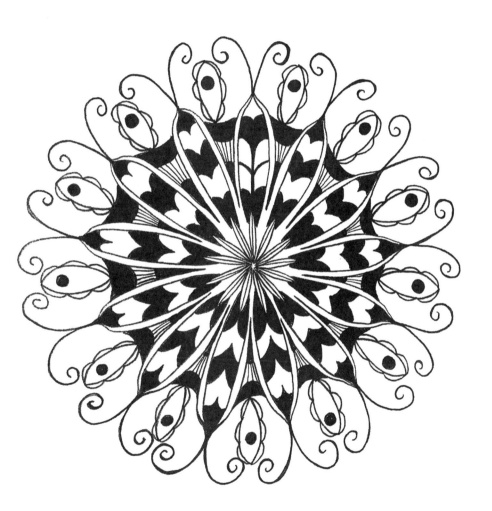

When I initiate and create touch that starts from my feet, my clients experience a fuller contact. Thinking of my hand, elbow or other working tool as the endpoint that delivers the earth's energy from my feet and through my body, both softens and deepens any technique. That depth is not just physical pressure; it is depth in the sense of profundity and richness of experience on many levels. I feel the difference too and my upper body can relax into perceiving more subtle cues from my client's tissue.

I especially enjoy using soothing, subtle rocking movements with firm deep pressure. Aimed to the deeper layers of the body and the nervous system, it is highly effective in reducing tension and pain due to misalignments, past lingering injuries, repetitive movements, traumatic experiences and chronic stress. Always moderated to be pleasurable, yet deep, most clients find this work to be both soothing and demanding in its intensity.

~ Carole Osborne ~
practicing the somatic arts and science since 1974
Author of Pre- and Perinatal Massage Therapy
and Deep Tissue Sculpting

Being able to be conscious of how you feel and to communicate your truth with honor and respect for yourself and for the other individual you are relating to. Maturing how to be an expert of yourself and not of the other person. Learning how to use the words in a positive way as they arevehicles of intention that create realities. Knowing that Healing is a slow and patient process, and how to give enough time and space so the self healing process can occur to its full possibility.

*~ **Maria Lucia Bittencourt Sauer** ~*
practicing spiritual massage since 1980

My years of experience in teaching massage have been one of the great gifts of my life, for I teach what I most need to be reminded of myself. The practice of awareness let's me be in the present moment with whomever I am touching and caring for, rather than the constant stream of thoughts in my head. In that space, my heart naturally opens to what ever is present. A nurturing connection is created between us; one that is rooted in acceptance, kindness, and empathy; that allows a softening, down to the cellular level. How lovely!

~ Carol A. Fitzgerald ~
practicing healing arts since 1983
Owner of Ceremonies With Heart and Meaning, Palo Alto, CA

My healing practices began in 1983. The way I bring presence to my work, is to notice my own body & breath. As I get in touch with this sensation, I feel more balanced and neutral, and can meet the person I'm working with from that place. Of course its not a fixed state, but a process that repeats many times.An idea that had a profound influence came from Monty Roberts (the original horse whisperer). He said that horses were "into pressure" animals, meaning that they move toward contact. The implications for bodywork were clear - instinctively we move towards pressure that is effective, and away from that which is intrusive. As my personal style developed, I found that I could achieve a deep yet non-intrusive connection to the aspect of the body I was working with by bringing the limb toward my pressure instead of "pushing" in.

My practice is called "Simply Grounded" - an umbrella term for the diverse practices I have chosen, and the way that ultimately they all align with this basic principle.

~ Rachel Johnson ~
practicing healing arts since 1983
Owner of Simply Grounded

212

When half the world is giving massage and half the
world is receiving massage, there will be peace on earth.

*~ **Debra Zager** ~*
practicing healing arts since 1992

It is a crazy, mad world out there! But what keeps me sane and grounded is my work in massage. I realize that I am very blessed to say this–my work brings me peace and joy. There have been many days that I've come into work stressed out or in tears from personal situations but as soon as I get to work there is a calming. Massage allows me to get out of my space and be present for others. It's a bit of an escape from reality. When I get out of my own body and connect with another person that is coming to me for healing-it's a complete shift. I always tell my clients that I am quiet during the treatment, which allows for me to concentrate on what their body may be needing and for them to be present in their own healing.

It is a joy to be able to extend my knowledge, skill and talent to those in need. The love that I put out always comes back to me, which is the true reward.

~ Amy Pontzloff ~
practicing healing arts since 1999
Owner of Lymphatic Face & Body Therapy, Redwood City, CA

As I am working with someone and I find an area of tension that is not releasing, I utilize what I call "mirroring." While applying a medium pressure, I close my eyes, take a deep breath, and find the same area and/or specific muscle that I'm massaging on my client in my own body, and I let go of any tension or holding there. When I release tension in a specific area of my own body I immediately feel a shift in the same area of my client's body!

~ Rakh Hargett ~
practicing healing arts since 2005

The one thing that is always present at the beginning of each massage session and that helps me stay grounded is the desire to honor the privilege that has been granted to me, to guide the client on the path of self-knowledge. Also, I used a technique call Entrainment which is a special process that happens when therapist and client are working together, with the breath, connected to each other with awareness. It is not synchronized breathing, where the therapist awkwardly tries to match the client's breathing. It is more natural than that, like when two people walking together naturally match each other's strides without thinking.

When the client breathes, I breathe, because both of us are enjoying the relaxation process. The human nervous system is ready, at birth to "entrain" with others. There is a deep feeling of safety and connectedness that happens when two people are breathing together. For me the most important skill you can learn as a massage therapist is the ability to pay attention to your own breath. The act of paying attention to your breath immediately brings your mind into the present moment, and it is only in the present moment that you can work with another person, in their present moment. so begin to breath...

~ Janie Sanabria ~
practicing healing arts since 2004

At the beginning of a session I usually make sure that I take some deeper breaths to slow me down. This reminds me of my intent and focus and allows my body to become more grounded and relaxed. And this can be an ongoing process throughout a session where I become aware of tension in my own self and then breathing can take me back down to where I need to be. In addition I was once told that the old Lomi Lomi masters, who were much more than just healers, were able to completely change their demeanor from warlike and aggressive to calm, peaceful and tranquil within the span of two breaths. Whether or not this is true I like visualizing this on occasion to calm myself down.

*~ **Casey Larrance** ~*
practicing healing arts since 1994

As I reverently place my hands upon the body, I say a silent prayer of gratitude & grace.

With clear communication including areas NOT to touch, areas of focus, and pressure preferences, I flow through the massage paying particular attention to my own body mechanics to avoid any injury. The best advice I can give a person who wants to perform any type of massage would be to "receive" as many massages as you can from a variety of therapists so in this way you can replicate those moves you liked best.

~ Mimi Stern ~
practicing healing arts since 1990

One of the most important things I learned early on in my career is the importance of how you, as a practitioner are feeling before you begin any massage. This is important due to the close connection you achieve with someone when using the power of touch. So before I begin a session, I take a few deep breaths all the way down into my abdomen, also known as diaphragmatic breathing. This type of breathing activates the parasympathetic branch of the autonomic nervous system which is the opposite of the fight or flight response. Within seconds of breathing this way, you will feel more calm, centered and relaxed. Then as you touch your client, through the process of entrainment, their breathing and vibration will change to match your own, allowing them to become more calm and to relax even deeper. This not only creates the conditions for an effective massage, but it also makes you more present which brings out the compassionate and nurturing aspects of yourself.

~ Darlene Marmer ~
practicing healing arts since 2001

A few key techniques I use to ground in and stay in the moment begins with taking notice to the rhythm and swell of my client's breathing as well as my own. Checking in with the breath helps me at times to determine their emotional state and how to better approach giving to this individual. To me, this is where the pace and flow of the session is decided. Once done, I then set my intentions upon the session. This is merely to identify what I would like to create for my client's massage. I do this by saying to myself, "I am a healer. My wish is to heal." And then it is so. Applying these methods can assist in placing a solid foundation moving forward into the massage session as well as keeping one centered throughout.

*~ **Robert L. Bard Jr.** ~*
practicing healing arts since 2002

Massage Therapy is holistic and communal. It's a healing partnership. My role as a massage therapist in the healing process is to take care of my whole being before engaging with others. It's important for me to maintain a healthy and constant level of inner awareness of my thoughts, emotions and body. Some helpful ways that help me become more self-aware is through meditation, either one-minute or thirty-minute, yoga, eating a delicious healthy meal, quiet walks, turning off the radio in the car, getting plenty of sleep, working in a quiet room, walking along the beach, cruising on my bike, listening to the dove outside my window, and more. As I listen and tune into my honest self, I can better navigate how to live a life of presence.

~ Upuia Ahkiong ~
practicing healing arts since 2002
Owner of Kua Body Studio, Los Altos, CA

Sometimes during sessions when I catch myself slouching and my mind wandering, I remind myself of a technique I heard in a yoga class once: *Pull your belly button into your spine.* As soon as I do this, my posture improves immediately – my chest opens up, the spine elongates and my hips tuck under me. It also brings me into the present moment, since it forces me to take a deep breath.

~ Heather Stillman ~
practicing healing arts since 1999

One of the most important blessings needed to massage is to be grounded in my work and sometimes to achieve this I hug a tree before sessions, carry a bit of dirt/sand in my shoes, or keep a small rock/quartz crystal in my pocket.

*~ **Anonymous** ~*
practicing healing arts since 2007

My massage mindset starts with the joy and serenity I have in my own life. I focus on this before I begin a session to ground me and remind me how blessed I am. I have compassion, strength and energy to give out today. If my mind drifts for any reason, I isolate one word : Gentle, Release, Peace, etc. and that returns me to the moment.

*~ **Mark Kinney** ~*
practicing healing arts since 1994
owner of World Class Education, Inc.

I ground myself before I begin a session, by planting my feet to the ground. I connect with the earth. I deepen my breath, engage three-part breathing and at this point it is important that I give my heart a smile. Really feeling my chest, collarbones, back rise and expand. Recognizing that the energy that will come through me to do the bodywork comes from the earth, air, fire and water, and energy released will flow back in to the earth, air, fire and water. This centers my mind body and spirit. The tool I find most useful during a massage session is my breath. Connecting with my breath allows me to stay present and receptive to what the clients needs are. In this way and others, breath is truly one of the most important tools in bodywork.

~ Emily Huber ~
practicing healing arts since 2003
Owner of Seeing Through the Hands Studio, Brooklyn, NY

Spinefulness cultivates the mind, body, spirit connection of yoga and brings it to daily life. Think of it as yoga anywhere, anytime. The power lies in one's ability to tap into the power the skeleton, relaxation, and breath at any time of day: at a traffic light, standing in line, walking. It's a presence practice- an awake meditation- that is practical for me as a mom of 3 kids because I don't need special circumstances to access Spinefulness: I just need an willingness to be open to possibility and my body. Spinefulness is borne out of relaxation.

~ Jean Couch ~
practicing Spinefulness since 1988
Certified by Noelle Perez of the Institute D'Aplomb, Paris
Founder of the Balance Center, Palo Alto, CA
Author of The Runner's Yoga Book

226

So you want to offer a massage to someone you know. Maybe you're new at this and you aren't quite sure just how to go about it. You aren't trained and don't feel all that confident, but you want to do well. Yes, it's good to know something about the anatomy of what you're touching. To be educated. To be smart and to use good technique. But in the absence of experience in these areas, consider that analytic thought will only take you so far, anyway. Know that you are not a disembodied mind, only thinking your way through this. Your body, with its own ways of knowing, knows something about these things. Be in this body of yours. Trust your senses. You are animal - a human animal, but animal nonetheless. Touch and sense and feel. Let your hands move in the ways they know to move. Trust your instinctual nature. Your hands know more than you think they do. They know how to touch with sensitivity, with curiosity and with compassionate intent, if you let them. They have life experience, and from that experience, they can begin to learn to touch another therapeutically. Just let them begin. Try being as a sculptor, kneading and molding tissues as you might sculpt modeling clay. Imagine you are softening, lengthening, guiding those muscles towards a flexible pliability. It's really pretty easy. Just relax into what you're doing, and be willing to not be perfect at first.

~Dr. Steven Stewart ~
practicing chiropractice since 1974
Owner of Stewert Chiropractic, Santa Cruz, CA

A Special Dedication to
Maria Lucia Bittencourt Sauer

The first time I met Maria was on a quiet afternoon in the Lodge at the Esalen Institute, where one can always find solitude or warm company along with hot tea and fresh bread. She struck me as warm and welcoming, and seemed to carry a slight air of secrecy or mystery – I couldn't quite put my finger on it, but I was curious about this woman. Then I learned from another patron that she taught spiritual massage. Well, my curiosity got that tickle it needed: I had to find out for myself!

She sat next to her co-teacher, Bo, in a low-lit room and behind her was what seemed to be some kind of makeshift shrine. The workshop participants and I sat around this mysterious woman and together we completed the human circle. In her quiet, unhurried voice, she explained that her shamanic lineage from Brazil, her work as a medium, her study with Chinese energetic work, and her Esalen massage had meshed, tangled into spiritual massage. Of course we participants had a lot of questions. One student in particular was firing question after question at her. Maria finally asked the student to hold on to her next question. There was a pause, then Maria said, "I would like to make sure I hear you right, digest your question and think it through before I answer. If I answer in a hurry, I might not be able to express myself clearly and correctly."

That was good medicine for me. I am surrounded by fast questions that demand instant answers, but how often do I really "digest" and listen? Listen to what is actually said, listen to my perception, and listen to my interpretation of what is being said. To listen is to be selfless and omnipresent. Maria's life

228

was dedicated to being present in the physical and the spiritual world. I feel blessed to have crossed paths with her, if only for a brief time. The lesson she passed on will most likely take me a lifetime to master.

Without the help and faith of my family and friends, this book would only live in my head. Thank you to Chade-Meng Tan and Steve Kettmann for encouraging me to write *OneBody Massage*. I want to acknowledge that without Steve Kettmann and Pete Danko's help on editing, *OneBody Massage* would probably only make sense to me. And a big thank you to these very special people for helping me to raise funds: Eric Gilmore, Abe Rahey, Steve Kettmann, Todd Johnston, Elisa Aldridge and Ryan Romsey.

Publisher's Note

At Wellstone Books we publish personal writing that is
not afraid to inspire and look to introduce fresh voices. *One-Body Massage* offers a grounding in massage and a window into
a world of greater connectivity, but it also shares Grace Ku's
personal story of turning away from a stressful computer job to
make a new life for herself as a massage therapist in Silicon Valley. We hope you enjoy both Grace's beautiful writing and her
stunning artwork on the cover and throughout the book. Grace
believes that through massage we can learn to communicate better with one another and move deeper into dialogue with our
own bodies. We can also help each other to fend off the warping
influence of stress, worry and fear, and bring joy into our days.
These are goals we support through other Wellstone Books titles
as well, such as *A Book of Walks* by Giants manager Bruce Bo-
chy, *a San Francisco Chronicle* bestseller that urges people to get
in regular long walks, and *Kiss the Sky* by Dusty Baker, the first
in our "Music That Changed My Life" series, all about Dusty's
lifelong love of music, focused on his weekend at the Monterey
Pop Festival in June 1967 and its lasting resonance.

~ *Steve Kettmann*

About the Wellstone Center in the Redwoods

Wellstone Books is the imprint of the Wellstone Center in the Redwoods, a writers retreat center in the Santa Cruz Mountains an hour and a half south of San Francisco hailed as "kind of like heaven" for writers in the *San Jose Mercury News* and named to *San Francisco Magazine's* "Best of the Bay" issue in 2003. WCR, founded in 2012 by Sarah Ringler and Steve Kettmann, offers weekend writing workshops, weeklong writing residences and monthlong writing fellowships. Visit our website at www.wellstoneredwoods.org for more information - or email us at info@wellstoneredwoods.org to apply. If you're in the Santa Cruz area, stop by our OpenMic night every Tuesday at 7 o'clock and read from a work in progress, play some music - or just sit and listen. We're at 858 Amigo Road in Soquel.